Behavior Change Log Book and Wellness Journal

Stephen L. Dodd

University of Florida

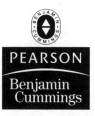

PEARSON

Benjamin Cummings

San Francisco   Boston   New York
Cape Town   Hong Kong   London   Madrid   Mexico City
Montreal   Munich   Paris   Singapore   Sydney   Tokyo   Toronto

Publisher: Daryl Fox

Senior Acquisitions Editor: Deirdre Espinoza

Project Editor: Susan Malloy

Assistant Editor: Alison Rodal

Managing Editor, Production: Deborah Cogan

Production Supervisor: Jane Brundage

Senior Marketing Manager: Sandra Lindelof

Manufacturing Buyer: Stacey Weinberger

Production Service and Composition: The Left Coast Group

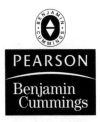

ISBN 0-8053-7844-8 (stand-alone version)
ISBN 0-8053-7936-3 (bundle version)
11 12 13 14—CRS—14 13 12 11 10
www.aw-bc.com

Table of Contents

This Behavior Change Log Book and Wellness Journal is intended as a tool to help you identify and change unhealthy behaviors; institute new, more healthy diet plans; develop and adhere to fitness prescriptions; reflect on health and wellness issues in journal exercises; and develop behavior change plans using short-term and lifelong Behavior Change Contracts.

Changing Behavior

This section of the Behavior Change Log Book will help you to modify problem behaviors. There are worksheets, assessments, and logs to aid in identifying target behaviors, developing strategies to overcoming them, and track your progress.

Lifestyle Assessment

The purpose of the following lifestyle assessment inventory is to raise your awareness of areas in your life that increase your risk of disease, injury, and possibly premature death. A key point to remember is that you have control over each of the lifestyle areas discussed.

Awareness is the first step in making change. After identifying the areas that require modification, use behavior modification techniques to bring about positive lifestyle changes.

Date _____

DIRECTIONS: Put a check by each statement that applies to you.

1. Physical Fitness

_____ I exercise for a minimum of 20 to 30 minutes at least 3 days per week.

_____ I play sports routinely (2 to 3 times per week).

_____ I walk for 15 to 30 minutes (3 to 7 days per week).

2. Body Fat

_____ There is no place on my body where I can pinch more than 1 inch of fat.

_____ I am satisfied with the way my body appears.

3. Stress Level

_____ I find it easy to relax.

_____ I rarely feel tense or anxious.

_____ I am able to cope with daily stresses better than most people.

4. Car Safety

_____ I have not had an auto accident in the past 4 years.

_____ I always use a seat belt when I drive.

_____ l rarely drive above the speed limit.

5. Sleep

_____ I always get 7 to 9 hours of sleep.

_____ l do not have trouble going to sleep.

_____ I generally do not wake up during the night.

6. Relationships

_____ I have a happy and satisfying relationship with my spouse or partner.

_____ I have a lot of close friends.

_____ I have a great deal of family love and support.

7. Diet

_____ I generally eat three balanced meals per day.

_____ I rarely overeat.

_____ I rarely eat large quantities of fatty foods and sweets.

8. Alcohol Use

_____ I consume fewer than two drinks per day.

_____ I never get intoxicated.

_____ I never drink and drive.

9. Tobacco Use

_____ I never smoke (cigarettes, pipe, cigars, etc.).

_____ I am not exposed to secondhand smoke on a regular basis.

_____ I do not use smokeless tobacco.

10. Drug Use

_____ I never use illicit drugs.

_____ I never abuse legal drugs such as diet or sleeping pills.

11. Safe Sex

_____ I always practice safe sex (e.g., always using condoms or being involved in a monogamous relationship).

EVALUATION

Individual areas: If you have fewer than three checks in categories 1 through 11, you can improve this area of your lifestyle.

Overall lifestyle: Add up your total number of checks. Scoring can be interpreted as follows:

23–29   Very healthy lifestyle

17–22   Average healthy lifestyle

16   Unhealthy lifestyle (needs improvement)

Common Target Behaviors

Four common target behaviors are examined below. If you think you are at risk for one or more of these behaviors it is important to start a behavior change program immediately.

Stress

Stress management is one of the five most important behaviors in promoting good health. Proper stress reduction techniques and behavior modifications are important to establish in order to reduce your risk of disease and accidents. In this section you will be able to assess the amount of stress in your life by answering the following questions.

Date _____

DIRECTIONS: The purpose of this stress index questionnaire is to increase your awareness of stress in your life. Answer *Yes* or *No* to each of the stress index questions. Circle your answer.

Yes   No   1. I have frequent arguments.

Yes   No   2. I often get upset at work.

Yes   No   3. I often have neck and/or shoulder pains due to anxiety/stress.

Yes   No   4. I often get upset when I stand in long lines.

Yes   No   5. I often get angry when I listen to the news or read the newspaper.

Yes   No   6. I do not have a sufficient amount of money for my needs.

Yes   No   7. I often get upset when driving.

Yes   No   8. At the end of a work day I often feel stress-related fatigue.

Yes   No   9. I have at least one constant source of stress/anxiety in my life
                  (e.g., conflict with boss, neighbor, mother-in-law, etc.).

Yes   No   10. I often have stress-related headaches.

Yes   No   11. I do not practice stress management techniques.

Yes   No   12. I rarely take time for myself.

Yes   No   13. I have difficulty in keeping my feelings of anger and hostility
                  under control.

Yes   No   14. I have difficulty in managing time wisely.

Yes   No   15. I often have difficulty sleeping.

Yes   No   16. I am generally in a hurry.

Yes   No   17. I usually feel that there is not enough time in the day to accomplish what I need to do.

Yes   No   18. I often feel that I am being mistreated by friends or associates.

Yes   No   19. I do not regularly perform physical activity.

Yes   No   20. I rarely get 7 to 9 hours of sleep per night.

EVALUATION

If you answered *Yes* to any of the questions you need to use some form of stress management techniques. Add your *Yes* answers and use the following scale to evaluate the level of stress in your life.

Number of *Yes* Answers

6–20   High stress

3–5   Average stress

0–2   Low stress

Using the Goal Log

If you're feeling too stressed the worksheets in this log book will help you develop a plan to combat those feelings. Use the Goal Log beginning on page 21 to track your progress; it may look something like this:

Target Behavior	Date	Goal	Goal Achieved?	What Happened?	New Strategy / New Goal
Excessive stress	12/1-12/8	Study for test w/o stressing out	Yes	When I felt stressed I took a 10 min jog & then went back to studying	Next time I get stressed studying I'll take a 5 min jog

Tobacco
Awareness of Smoking Dangers

Date _____

DIRECTIONS: Answer the following questions *True* or *False* to test your knowledge of the dangers of smoking. Circle your answer.

T   F   1. Smoking increases your risk of lung cancer and heart disease.

T   F   2. Smoking is the most common avoidable cause of death.

T   F   3. Heavy smokers are 15–25 times more likely to die of cancer than nonsmokers.

T   F   4. Smoking soothes the throat and lungs by relaxing the cilia.

T   F   5. Smoking causes an increased risk of oral, pancreatic, and bladder cancer.

T   F   6. The average life expectancy for a chronic smoker is 7 years shorter than for a nonsmoker.

T   F   7. Smoking a pipe is less harmful than smoking cigarettes.

T   F   8. Pipes, cigarettes, and smokeless tobacco increase your risk of oral cancer.

T   F   9. Secondhand smoke is carcinogenic (cancer causing).

T   F   10. Chewing tobacco is harmless because there is no smoke to get into your lungs.

T   F   11. Smoking is not addictive.

EVALUATION

Questions 4, 7, 10, and 11 are *False*, all of the others are *True*. If you smoke or use tobacco you are at risk.

Smoking Cessation

Now that you are aware of the dangers and harmful effects of smoking, it's time to make a conscious decision to stop. There are three phases to a smoking cessation program: the preparation phase, the cessation phase, and the maintenance phase.

Date _____

DIRECTIONS: Complete the following sections to help form your smoking cessation strategy and to assist you through these phases.

I. Preparation Phase

1. I have a strong desire to stop smoking.

    a. yes

    b. no

2. I smoke because _____ .

    a. of peers or social situations

    b. of nicotine addiction

    c. I think it looks cool

    d. other

II. Cessation Phase

Smoking Cessation Contract

1. I _____ agree to stop smoking beginning on _____ .
           (name)   (date)

2. My short term goal is to stop smoking on _____ .
                                                 (date)

3. My long term goal is *to remain smoke free for life*.

4. I will avoid situations such as _____ , _____ , and _____ that may hinder my smoking cessation.

5. I will report my progress to _____ and _____ on a regular basis.

6. If tempted to smoke, I will _____ and/or _____ instead.

   Signed _____   Date _____

   Witness _____   Date _____

III. Maintenance Phase

1. In order to ensure that I will remain smoke free, I will have _____ ,

   _____ , and _____ as my support group.

2. I will avoid _____ , _____ , and _____ situations.

3. I will continue to educate myself on the dangers of smoking by _____ ,

   _____ , and _____ .

Using the Goal Log

If you are addicted to cigarettes or other tobacco products the worksheets in this log book can help you design a plan to break your addiction. Use the Goal Log beginning on page 21 to track your progress; it may look something like this:

Target Behavior	Date	Goal	Goal Achieved?	What Happened?	New Strategy / New Goal
Smoking	*3/7-3/21*	*Cut down to 1/2 pack per week by 3/21*	*No*	*Smoked a lot of cigarettes at a party*	*Next time I'm at a party I'll try to avoid being around people who smoke*

STIs

Every year twelve million people in the United States are infected by one or more sexually transmitted infections (STIs). STIs are generally spread through sexual contact but can also be contracted through shared needles or blood. There is no cure for AIDS or herpes, and although treatment methods exist for many other STIs, prevention is clearly the best approach.

Date _____

DIRECTIONS: Answer the following questions to assess your risk for contracting STIs. Circle your answer.

Yes   No   1. I engage in sexual activity.

Yes   No   2. I have more than one sexual partner.

Yes   No   3. I use drugs or alcohol.

Yes   No   4. I engage in oral sex.

Yes   No   5. I share hypodermic needles or other devices with which blood exchange may occur (e.g., razors, ear-piercing instruments, tattoo instruments).

Yes   No   6. I do not practice safe sex (e.g., using a condom).

Yes   No   7. I do not have a yearly physical and routine check-ups.

EVALUATION

If you answered *Yes* to any of these questions you may be at risk for contracting an STI.

Using the Goal Log

If you feel you are at risk for an STI you should begin practicing safe sex and avoid alcohol, drugs, or other substances that may promote unsafe behavior. Visit a doctor or other health care provider for STI testing and information on ways to protect yourself. To maintain a program that keeps you free of risk use this log book to develop goals and strategies. Use the Goal Log beginning on page 21 to track your progress; it may look something like this:

Target Behavior	Date	Goal	Goal Achieved?	What Happened?	New Strategy / New Goal
Excessive drinking and potential exposure to STIs	*10/8*	*Avoid drinking in potentially risky situations*	*Yes*	*When tempted to get drunk I thought about the repercussions of irresponsible behavior*	*Now I will try to avoid risky situations completely*

Cancer

Cancer is the second leading cause of death in the United States, and lifestyle habits such as smoking, eating high-fat diets, drinking excessively, and sunbathing are all contributors to an increased risk of cancer.

Date _____

DIRECTIONS: Answer the following questions *Yes* or *No* to determine your risk. Circle your answer.

Yes   No   1. Do you consume a high-fat diet (e.g., >30% total calorie intake)?

Yes   No   2. Is your diet low in fiber?

Yes   No   3. Do you consume an excessive amount of alcohol?

Yes   No   4. Do you regularly eat smoked foods?

Yes   No   5. Are you exposed to environmental carcinogens (cancer-causing agents)?

Yes   No   6. Do you use tobacco products or breathe secondhand smoke?

Yes   No   7. Are you obese?

Yes   No   8. Do you have a family history of cancer?

Yes   No   9. Is your skin regularly exposed to excessive sunlight?

Yes   No   10. Do you have a fair complexion?

EVALUATION

Answering *Yes* to any of the questions means that you should modify your lifestyle to reduce your risk of cancer.

Using the Goal Log

Reduce your risk of cancer by maintaining a healthy diet, exercising regularly, avoiding carcinogens, and limiting excess exposure to the sun. For further information, see your text. Use this log book to develop strategies and goals for modifying your behavior. Use the Goal Log beginning on page 21 to track your progress; it may look something like this:

Target Behavior	Date	Goal	Goal Achieved?	What Happened?	New Strategy / New Goal
Sunbathing w/o sunscreen	*6/17*	*Use at least SPF 15 when outdoors; reapply regularly*	*No*	*Forgot to bring sunscreen to the beach*	*Now I'll keep the sunscreen in my car so that I'll have it when I drive to the ocean*

Target Behaviors

Date _____

DIRECTIONS: In the following spaces list five behaviors that you want to change. Examples of target behaviors include smoking, eating unhealthy foods, and not exercising regularly.

Target Behaviors:

1. _____

2. _____

3. _____

4. _____

5. _____

Choose the target behavior you feel the most strongly about changing and use the following worksheets and logs to help you modify that behavior. Once you've succeeded in changing that behavior pick another one to work on.

Identifying Addictive Behaviors

Date _____

DIRECTIONS: To help you decide if your target behavior is addictive answer the following questions, substituting your target behavior in the blanks. Circle your answer.

Yes No 1. Do you _____ alone?

Yes No 2. Do you _____ on a regular basis?

Yes No 3. When you are stressed do you _____?

Yes No 4. Do you crave _____ at any time of the day?

Yes No 5. Are you influenced by others to _____?

Yes No 6. Does your _____ impair your job performance or ability to engage in daily activitites?

Yes No 7. Does your _____ cause you to use poor judgement?

Yes No 8. Do you lie to friends or family about how much or how often you _____?

Yes No 9. Have you tried unsuccessfully to cut down on _____?

EVALUATION

If you answer *Yes* to any of these questions, you may be addicted. If this addiction affects your health (e.g., smoking) you should talk with a physician or other health care provider.

Health Costs and Benefits
of My Target Behavior

To better understand the importance of your behavior change, it is important to recognize the harmful effects of your present target behavior and the positive effects of quitting that behavior.

Some negative effects of my target behavior include:

1. _____

2. _____

3. _____

4. _____

Some positive effects of my behavior change include:

1. _____

2. _____

3. _____

4. _____

Monitoring Behavior

In order to better understand why and when you engage in your target behavior, it is important to monitor that behavior.

DIRECTIONS: Use the following table to monitor your target behavior for at least 3 days.

Date	How long did it last? Intensity?	When did it occur?	Where did it occur?

What else were you doing?	Other influences?	Your thoughts and feelings about it?

Setting Goals and Choosing Rewards

Now that you have examined your current behavior you can begin to plan a change in your future actions. An important part of this plan will be choosing specific goals and rewards.

Goals

Whatever your target behavior is, there are several key points to remember when establishing goals.

1. Establish achievable goals.

2. Put goals in writing and place them where you can see them everyday.

3. Establish both short- and long-term goals.

4. Establish goals that are measurable.

5. Set target dates for achieving goals.

6. After you achieve a goal, establish another achievable goal.

7. Reward yourself after achievement of a goal.

Rewards

It is important to reward yourself for accomplishments and goals that you have met. Rewards should be things that you may not always get to do, but things that you enjoy doing. They should be relatively inexpensive and accessible, and they should not be anything that reinforces the behavior you are trying to change. Rewards for someone trying to lose weight might be shopping or taking a walk on the beach, rather then going out to eat or eating sweets.

DIRECTIONS: Use the paragraph below to assist you in setting goals by filling in the appropriate responses in the blanks.

My goal is to _____
                                    (long-term goal)

The short-term goals I have established to help me achieve my long-term goal are

_____ , _____ and _____

The deadlines that I have set for myself to achieve these goals and the rewards I will receive upon completing them are as follows:

_____	_____	_____
(short-term goal 1)	(date)	(reward)
_____	_____	_____
(short-term goal 2)	(date)	(reward)
_____	_____	_____
(short-term goal 3)	(date)	(reward)

My deadline to achieve my long-term goal is _____ The reward I will give
                                                    (date)

myself upon completion is _____
                                (reward)

Challenges to Behavior Change and Strategies to Overcome Them

After establishing your short-term and long-term goals for behavior change, you will find that there will be many distractions and challenges that may hinder your progress. In order to overcome these challenges, you must develop strategies to counteract them. The Examining Attitudes worksheet will help to uncover some potential difficulties and methods for dealing with them. Upon overcoming a challenge, you should reward yourself for a job well done.

Example of Strategies

Target Behavior Change: Weight Loss

Susan has decided that she wants to lose weight. She has established a program for herself that includes eating healthy, proportionate meals every day and exercising at least five days a week. Susan has been invited to a Super Bowl party that includes a big barbeque with lots of food, chips, sweets, and beer. She really wants to go to the party but does not want to break her weight loss program. What should she do?

Strategies

Some suggestions for Susan might be to eat a healthy meal before the barbeque so that when she arrives she is not hungry, and possibly not as tempted, as if she arrived with an empty stomach. Susan might also bring a plate of vegetables and low-fat dip to share with the guests. If she is hungry, she should stick to the healthier snack that she brought. Susan might also want to socialize with guests in an area away from the food. After the party, she should reward herself for overcoming the temptations by engaging in an activity that she enjoys.

Examining Attitudes and Creative Strategies

Understanding your attitudes and feelings about your target behavior will help you better understand why you engage in that behavior and what might prevent you from changing it. This knowledge will allow you to create effective strategies.

DIRECTIONS: Fill in the blanks with the appropriate answers.

I engage in _____ because _____
          (target behavior)

_____

I am most tempted to _____ when _____
               (target behavior)

_____

I have not quit _____ because _____
        (target behavior)

_____

_____ is difficult for me because _____
   (behavior goal)

_____

_____

I feel that _____ would help me to achieve _____
        (strategy 1)   (behavior goal)

because _____

I feel that _____ would help me to achieve _____
        (strategy 2)   (behavior goal)

because _____

I feel that _____ would help me to achieve _____
        (strategy 3)   (behavior goal)

because _____

Once I achieve _____ I can stick to it by _____
          (behavior goal)   (maintenance strategy)

_____

Behavior Change Contract

DIRECTIONS: Complete the following behavior change contract for your target behavior. Choose a friend or peer as a witness.

I _____ agree to _____
(name)   (behavior change)

_____.

I will begin on _____ and plan to reach my goal of _____
(start date)   (final goal)

_____

by _____.
(final target date)

In order to make my goals more attainable I have devised a list of short-term goals.

_____	_____	_____
(short-term goal 1)	(target date)	(reward)
(short-term goal 2)	(target date)	(reward)
(short-term goal 3)	(target date)	(reward)

I have identified challenges to my behavior change and have developed the following strategies to overcome them.

_____	_____
(challenge 1)	(strategy 1)
(challenge 2)	(strategy 2)
(challenge 3)	(strategy 3)

By signing this contract I have made a commitment to changing my behavior and I have

had _____ to witness my contract.
(witness)

_____   _____
(your signature)   (witness signature)

Goal Log

Use this log to track your progress. If you have set daily goals, use the log daily; if you have set weekly goals, use the log weekly.

Target Behavior	Date	Goal	Goal Achieved?	What Happened?	New Strategy / New Goal

Target Behavior	Date	Goal	Goal Achieved?	What Happened?	New Strategy / New Goal

Target Behavior	Date	Goal	Goal Achieved?	What Happened?	New Strategy / New Goal

Target Behavior	Date	Goal	Goal Achieved?	What Happened?	New Strategy / New Goal

Target Behavior	Date	Goal	Goal Achieved?	What Happened?	New Strategy / New Goal

Nutrition and Weight Management

Nutrition and weight management are critical aspects of a healthy lifestyle. A change in your lifestyle that emphasizes proper nutrition and weight management can lower your risk of disease and improve your health and well-being. The following section will help you get started.

Nutrition

For fitness and wellness, there is nothing more important than nutrition. Nutrients provide energy and the essential molecules necessary for shaping and operating the body's systems. The adage is true, "You are what you eat."

The "eating right pyramid" (below) is a great place to begin planning a new diet.

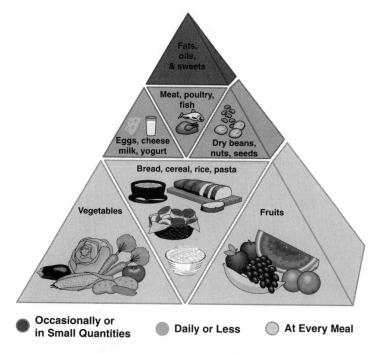

Source: Donatelle, R. J., and L. G. Davis, *Access to Health*, 2002. Copyright © 2002. Reprinted by permission of Benjamin Cummings.

The basic diet should consist mainly of the foods on the lower two tiers of the eating right pyramid, and decreasing amounts of the foods higher up. Follow the suggestions below to make a quick and effective improvement in your diet.

- Fresh, frozen, dried, or canned vegetables all provide important nutrients.

- Choose a variety of vegetable colors and types; dark-green leafy vegetables, bright orange fruits and vegetables, and cooked or dried peas and beans are all good options.

- Consume only the amount of calories that you need to maintain body weight.

- It is not difficult to get the protein you need (10–15% of calories). Make sure to get all the essential amino acids each day. For vegetarians this means combining a variety of vegetables and grains to form complementary proteins.

- Reduce fat consumption. Make sure that no more than 30% of calories per day come from fat.

- Reduce simple sugars such as desserts, candy, and ice cream.

- Last, but not least, consume lots of water. This is especially true if you exercise routinely. Keep water available and drink water with meals.

Portion Sizes

When figuring out your daily nutrient intake, you have to take into account *how much* you are eating. You may be confused by how much an ounce, a cup, or a "medium" apple is. The list below gives you a general idea of how to relate these measures to what's on your plate.

- 1 medium apple
  - the size of a baseball

- 1 teaspoon (5 ml)
  - the volume of your little finger

- 1 ounce (28 g)
  - 1 slice of bread or cheese (sandwich size)
  - enough nuts to cover the palm of your hand
  - $1/8$ of a medium apple

- 2 ounces (56 g)
  - $1/4$ of a medium apple
  - $1/2$ cup of peanut butter

- 4 ounces (112 g)
  - 1 fish filet
  - 1 small orange
  - 1 hamburger patty

- $1/2$ cup (118 ml)
  - a handful of dried fruit
  - a water cooler cup

- 1 cup (236 ml)
  - about the volume of a baseball
  - volume of a standard light bulb

Diet Assessment

Use the following tables to record your daily dietary habits for 3 days (try to include week-days and weekend days). Tables listing the nutritional values of common and fast foods appear on pages 49–69. The eating right pyramid and the recommended allowances will help you determine where changes in your diet need to be made.

* Your daily kcal requirement is determined by your daily caloric expenditure (see page 41). You can create a calorie deficit to lose weight, but it should be no more than 500kcal/day.

† Your daily protein intake should be _____ x 0.36g/lb = _____ g.
(body weight in lbs)

Pregnant women should add an additional 15g daily and lactating women should add 20g daily.

‡ Calcium: Males and females 9–18 years old need 1300mg, 19–50 years old need 1000mg, and 51 and older need 1200mg.

§ Iron: Males 9–13 years old and 19 and older need 8mg, 14–18 years old need 11mg.
Females 9–13 years old and 51 and older need 8mg, 14–18 years old need 15mg, 19–50 years old need 18mg, pregnant (any age) need 27mg, and lactating need 9mg if over 19 years old and 10mg if under.

DAY ONE Food	Vegetable Servings	Breads and Cereals Servings	Fruit Servings	Dairy Servings	Meats and Protein Servings	Calories (kcals)	Protein (gm)	Carbohydrate (g)	Fiber (g)	Fat (g)	Fat % (kcal)	Saturated Fat (g)	Cholestorol (mg)	Sodium (mg)	Vitamin A (ug)	Vitamin C (mg)	Calcium (mg)	Iron (mg)
TOTALS																		
Recommended	3–5	6–11	2–4	2–3	2–3	See note *	See note †	>58% of diet	30% of diet	<30% of diet		<10% of diet	<300	3000	700–900	65–90	See note ‡	See note §

DAY TWO Food	Vegetable Servings	Breads and Cereals Servings	Fruit Servings	Dairy Servings	Meats and Protein Servings	Calories (kcals)	Protein (gm)	Carbohydrate (g)	Fiber (g)	Fat (g)	Fat % (kcal)	Saturated Fat (g)	Cholestorol (mg)	Sodium (mg)	Vitamin A (ug)	Vitamin C (mg)	Calcium (mg)	Iron (mg)
TOTALS																		
Recommended	3–5	6–11	2–4	2–3	2–3	See note *	See note †	>58% of diet	30% of diet	<30% of diet		<10% of diet	<300	3000	700–900	65–90	See note ‡	See note §

DAY THREE Food	Vegetable Servings	Breads and Cereals Servings	Fruit Servings	Dairy Servings	Meats and Protein Servings	Calories (kcals)	Protein (gm)	Carbohydrate (g)	Fiber (g)	Fat (g)	Fat % (kcal)	Saturated Fat (g)	Cholestorol (mg)	Sodium (mg)	Vitamin A (ug)	Vitamin C (mg)	Calcium (mg)	Iron (mg)
TOTALS																		
Recommended	3–5	6–11	2–4	2–3	2–3	See note *	See note †	>58% of diet	30% of diet	<30% of diet		<10% of diet	<300	3000	700–900	65–90	See note ‡	See note §

Nutrition Plan

After studying my 3-day assessment I see that my diet is lacking in the following nutrients or food groups:

_____

I can increase my intake of these nutrients/food groups by eating the following healthy, low-fat, low-sugar foods:

_____

_____

After studying my 3-day assessment I see that my diet consists of too much of the following nutrients/food groups:

_____

I can decrease my intake of these nutrients/food groups by cutting out unnecessary foods such as:

_____

_____

Fill out the behavior change contract on page 45 when you are ready to begin your new nutrition plan.

Nutrition Log

Use this log after you have developed your new nutrition plan and record what you eat each day. It will help you assess how well you are sticking to your plan. For detailed information on the nutritional content of your diet, you can enter the foods from your log into NutriFit software and receive a complete nutrient breakdown.

TIP: *Record things like where you ate, what else you were doing, and your thoughts and feelings while eating in the Comments column.*

Time of Day	Meal or Snack?	Food	Food Group	Serving Size	Comments

Date _____ Day of Week _____

Time of Day	Meal or Snack?	Food	Food Group	Serving Size	Comments

Date _____ Day of Week _____

Time of Day	Meal or Snack?	Food	Food Group	Serving Size	Comments

Date _____   Day of Week _____

Time of Day	Meal or Snack?	Food	Food Group	Serving Size	Comments

Date _____   Day of Week _____

Time of Day	Meal or Snack?	Food	Food Group	Serving Size	Comments

Date _____ Day of Week _____

Time of Day	Meal or Snack?	Food	Food Group	Serving Size	Comments

Date _____ Day of Week _____

Time of Day	Meal or Snack?	Food	Food Group	Serving Size	Comments

Weight Management

Maintaining a healthy body weight is important in reducing your risk for disease and injury. Several key points to a healthy weight-management program are listed below. Keep these in mind as you develop your weight management plan.

1. Determine your present weight. Calculate your body mass index and determine if you really need to lose or gain weight.

2. Make your goals realistic. Don't try to accomplish too much, too fast. Set short-term goals that you can accomplish followed by long-term goals that focus on your overall plan.

3. Eat healthy. Move away from higher calorie or processed foods and substitute lower calorie, unprocessed foods.

4. Start an exercise program. Exercise burns calories, build muscles, helps regulate blood sugar levels and appetite, reduces nervous tension, helps you cope with stress, and improves mood and self-image.

5. Recruit your friends to help. A partner makes your program easier to follow.

6. Work on your psychological well-being. Relaxing and having fun may help you resist some of the emotional drive to overeat.

7. Don't be upset by plateaus or setbacks. There will be times when you don't seem to be making progress. Or, there may be problems that prevent you from following your plan. Don't get discouraged! Problems will happen, and you must be persistent and continue your program.

8. Make long-term goals. These are hard to pursue because you get little feedback in the short-term. Use short-term goals to help you realize the long-term goals.

9. Remember, health is the ultimate goal. Weight loss may be your focus, but if your health suffers your long-term goal has not been achieved.

10. Log your progress. Maintaining this log book will be an essential part of your plan to record and achieve your goals.

Determining Ideal Body Weight and Estimating Daily Caloric Expenditure

Computation of Ideal Body Weight Using Body Mass Index (BMI)

The BMI uses the metric system. Therefore, you must express your weight in kilograms (1 kilogram = 2.2 pounds) and your height in meters (1 inch = 0.0254 meters).

STEP 1: COMPUTE YOUR BMI

BMI = body weight (kg)/(height in meters)^2

Your BMI = _____

STEP 2: CALCULATE YOUR IDEAL BODY WEIGHT BASED ON BMI*

The ideal BMI is 21.9 to 22.4 for men and 21.3 to 22.1 for women. The formula for computing ideal body weight using BMI is

ideal body weight (kilograms) = desired BMI x (height in meters)^2

Consider the following example as an illustration of the computation of ideal body weight. A woman who weighs 60 kilograms and is 1.5 meters tall computes her BMI to be 26.7. Her ideal BMI is between 21.9 and 22.4; therefore, her ideal body weight range is

ideal body weight = 21.9 x 2.25 = 49.3 kilograms

ideal body weight = 22.4 x 2.25 = 50.4 kilograms

Now complete this calculation using your values for BMI.

My ideal body weight range using the BMI method is _____ to _____ kilograms.

Note: *BMI may not be a good method to determine ideal body weight for a highly muscled individual.*

Estimating Daily Caloric Expenditure and the Caloric Deficit Required to Lose 1 Pound of Fat per Week.

PART A. ESTIMATION OF DAILY CALORIC EXPENDITURE BASED ON BODY WEIGHT AND PHYSICAL ACTIVITY

Date _____

To compute your estimated daily caloric expenditure, multiply your body weight in pounds by the calories per pound that corresponds to your activity level.

Activity Level	Description	Calories per Pound of Body Weight Expended during a 24-hour Period
1	Very sedentary (restricted movement, such as a patient confined to a house)	13
2	Sedentary (most U.S. citizens; light work or office job)	14
3	Moderate activity (many college students; some daily activity and weekend recreation)	15
4	Very physically active (vigorous activity at least 3–4 times/week)	16
5	Competitive athlete (daily activity in high-energy sport)	17–18

Estimated daily caloric expenditure = _____ calories/day.

PART B. CALCULATION OF CALORIC INTAKE REQUIRED TO PROMOTE 1 POUND PER WEEK OF WEIGHT LOSS

Recall that 1 pound of fat contains approximately 3500 calories. Therefore, a negative caloric balance of 500 calories/day will result in a weight loss of 1 pound per week. Use the following formula to compute your daily caloric intake that would result in a daily caloric deficit of 500 calories.

estimated daily caloric expenditure – 500 calories (deficit) = daily caloric intake needed to produce a 500-calorie deficit

In the space provided, compute your daily caloric intake needed to produce a weight loss of 1 pound per week.

_____ (estimated caloric expenditure) –

_____–500_____ (caloric deficit) =

_____ (target daily caloric intake)

Weight Training and Exercise

- For those who want to gain weight, it is important to remember that eating more calories will cause an increase in body fat. Of course, this is undesirable. The only healthy way to gain body weight is to add muscle mass. This can only be accomplished through weight training.

- Exercise must play a role in any weight management program. Exercise increases caloric expenditure both during and long after completing a workout. The table below provides information on the energy costs for selected sporting activities.

Energy Costs for Selected Sporting Activities

Sport	Cal/min./kg
Archery (American Round)	0.0412
Bowling (with three other bowlers)	0.0471
Golf (playing in a foursome)	0.0559
Walking (17-min. mile on a grass surface)	0.0794
Cycling (6.4-min. mile)	0.0985
Canoeing (15-min. mile)	0.1029
Swimming (50-yd./min.)	0.1333
Running (10-min. mile)	0.1471
Cycling (5-min. mile)	0.1559
Handball (singles)	0.1603
Skipping rope (80 turns/rnin.)	0.1655
Running (8-min. mile)	0.1856
Running (6-min. mile)	0.2350

Source: Physical Fitness, 5th ed., by Bud Getchell et al. Copyright © 1992 by Benjamin Cummings.

Setting Goals

It is important to set goals for your new weight management program. Refer to the Changing Behaviors section of this log book for guidelines on setting useful short-term and long-term goals. The information below may help you in forming goals for your weight management program.

My current weight is _____

I would like to weigh _____

My current daily caloric intake is _____

My target caloric intake is _____

In order to attain my target caloric intake I will create a caloric difference of _____

by modifying my diet and a caloric difference of _____ through exercise.

Behavior Change Contract

DIRECTIONS: Complete the following behavior change contract for your weight management program/nutrition plan. Choose a friend or peer as a witness.

I _____ agree to _____
              (name)   (behavior change)

_____.

I will begin on _____ and plan to reach my goal of _____
                (start date)   (final goal)

_____

by _____.
     (final target date)

In order to make my goals more attainable I have devised a list of short-term goals.

(short-term goal 1)	(target date)	(reward)
(short-term goal 2)	(target date)	(reward)
(short-term goal 3)	(target date)	(reward)

I have identified challenges to my behavior change and have developed the following strategies to overcome them.

(challenge 1)	(strategy 1)
(challenge 2)	(strategy 2)
(challenge 3)	(strategy 3)

By signing this contract I have made a commitment to changing my behavior and I have

had _____ to witness my contract.
            (witness)

(your signature)	(witness signature)

Weight Management Log

DIRECTIONS: Use the following log to track your progress.

		ENTER						CALCULATE		
		Weight* (lbs)		Food (kcal)		Exercise (kcal)		Weight Diff.	Food Diff.	Exercise Diff.
Date	Day	Goal	Today	Goal	Today	Goal	Today	(lbs)	(kcal)	(kcal)

*Measure body weight weekly.

		ENTER						CALCULATE		
		Weight* (lbs)		Food (kcal)		Exercise (kcal)		Weight Diff.	Food Diff.	Exercise Diff.
Date	Day	Goal	Today	Goal	Today	Goal	Today	(lbs)	(kcal)	(kcal)

*Measure body weight weekly.

		ENTER							CALCULATE		
		Weight* (lbs)		Food (kcal)		Exercise (kcal)		Weight Diff. (lbs)	Food Diff. (kcal)	Exercise Diff. (kcal)
Date	Day	Goal	Today	Goal	Today	Goal	Today			

*Measure body weight weekly.

Nutritional Content of Common Foods and Beverages

The following table of nutrient values it taken from the EvaluEat diet analysis software that is a supplement to this text. The foods in the table shown here are just a fraction of the foods provided in the software. When using the software, you can quickly find these by entering the EvaluEat code in the search field. Values are obtained from the USDA Nutrient Database for Standard References, Release 16. A "0" indicates that nutrient value is determined to be zero; a blank space indicates that nutrient information is not available.

Amt = serving amount

Wt = weight

Ener = energy

Prot = protein

Carb = carbohydrate

Fiber = dietary fiber

Fat = total fat

Sat = saturated fat

Chol = cholesterol

Calc = calcium

Iron = iron

Sodi = sodium

EvaluEat Code	Food Name	Amount	Wt (g)	Ener (kcal)
Grains				
18001	Bagel, Plain/Onion/Poppy/Sesame, enriched	1 bagel (4" dia)	89	244.75
18013	Biscuit, Plain or Buttermilk, refrig dough, baked, reduced fat	1 biscuit (2-1/4" dia)	21	62.79
18035	Bread, Mixed Grain/7-Grain/Whole Grain	1 slice, large	32	80
18041	Bread, Pita, White, enriched	1 pita, large (6-1/2" dia)	60	165
18042	Bread, Pita, Whole Wheat	1 pita, large (6-1/2" dia)	64	170.24
18055	Bread, Wheat, reduced kcal	1 slice	23	45.54
18069	Bread, White, commercially prep, crumbs/cubes/slices	1 slice	25	66.5
18057	Bread, White, reduced kcal	1 slice	23	47.61
43100	Breakfast bars, oats, sugar, raisins, coconut (include granola bar)	1 cup	186	863.04
8053	Cereal, 100% Bran (wheat bran & barley)	.333 cup (1 NLEA serving)	29	83.23
8037	Cereal, Granola (oats & wheat germ) homemade	1 cup	122	597.8
8284	Cereal, Low Fat Granola with Raisins/Kellogg	.667 cup (1 NLEA serving)	55	201.3
8180	Cereal, Oats, Regular/Quick/Instant, ckd w/salt	1 cup	234	145.08
8157	Cereal, Wheat, Puffed, fortified	1 cup	12	43.68
8147	Cereal, Wheat, Shredded, large biscuit	2 biscuits (1 NLEA serving)	46	156.4
18620	Cracker, Original Premium Saltine Crackers/Nabisco	1 serving	14	58.8
18621	Cracker, Ritz/Nabisco	1 serving	16	78.72
18235	Cracker, Whole Wheat	10 Triscuit Bits	10	44.3
18258	English Muffin, Plain/Sourdough, enriched	1 muffin	57	133.95
20029	Grain, Couscous, ckd	1 cup, cooked	157	175.84
20037	Grain, Rice, Brown, Long grain, ckd	1 cup	195	216.45
20345	Grain, Rice, White, Long grain, enriched, ckd w/salt	1 cup	158	205.4
22005	Macaroni and Cheese Dinner, Kraft Original Flavor, unprepared	1 NLEA Serving (makes about 1 cup prepared)	70	259
20100	Macaroni, enriched, cooked	1 cup elbow shaped	140	197.4
18274	Muffin, Blueberry, commercially prep	1 medium	113	313.01
18279	Muffin, Corn, commercially prep	1 medium	113	344.65
20113	Noodles, Chinese, Chow Mein	1 cup	45	237.15
20110	Noodles, Egg, enriched, ckd w/salt	1 cup	160	212.8
18293	Pancakes, Plain, homemade	1 pancake (4" dia)	38	86.26
20121	Pasta, Spaghetti, enriched, ckd w/o salt	1 cup	140	197.4
43572	Popcorn, microwave, low fat and sodium	1 cup	148	634.92
18349	Roll, French	1 roll	38	105.26
18350	Roll, Hamburger/HotDog, Plain	1 roll	43	119.97
19015	Snack, Granola Bar, Hard, Plain	1 bar (1 oz)	28	131.88
19020	Snack, Granola Bar, Soft, Plain	1 bar (1 oz)	28	124.04
19034	Snack, Popcorn, air-popped	1 cup	8	30.56
19051	Snack, Rice Cake, brown rice, Plain	2 cakes	18	69.66
22901	Tortellini, pasta with cheese filling	1 cup	236	724.52
18449	Tortilla, Corn, w/o salt, ready to cook	1 tortilla, medium (approx 6" dia)	26	57.72
18364	Tortilla, Flour, ready-to-cook	1 tortilla medium (approx 6" dia)	46	149.5
18365	Waffle, Plain/Buttermilk, frozen, ready-to-heat	1 waffle square	39	97.89

Prot (g)	Carb (g)	Fiber (g)	Fat (g)	Sat (g)	Chol (g)	Calc (mg)	Iron (mg)	Sodi (mg)
9.345	47.526	2.047	1.424	0.196	0	65.86	3.168	475.26
1.638	11.634	0.399	1.092	0.272	0	3.99	0.649	304.71
3.2	14.848	2.048	1.216	0.258	0	29.12	1.11	155.84
5.46	33.42	1.32	0.72	0.1	0	51.6	1.572	321.6
6.272	35.2	4.736	1.664	0.262	0	9.6	1.958	340.48
2.093	10.028	2.76	0.529	0.079	0	18.4	0.681	117.53
1.91	12.653	0.6	0.822	0.179	0	37.75	0.935	170.25
2.001	10.189	2.231	0.575	0.126	0	21.62	0.734	104.19
18.228	124.062	5.766	32.736	23.603	0	111.6	5.915	517.08
3.683	22.678	8.294	0.609	0.087	0	22.04	8.1	120.93
18.141	64.599	10.492	29.719	5.535	0	95.16	5.185	26.84
4.4	44	2.75	2.75	0.825	0	23.1	1.65	135.3
6.084	25.272	3.978	2.34	0.421	0	18.72	1.591	374.4
1.764	9.552	0.528	0.144	0.024	0	3.36	3.804	0.48
5.235	36.138	5.336	1.104	0.207	0	20.24	1.509	5.52
1.526	9.954	0.364	1.428	0.259	0	27.02	0.727	177.8
1.152	10.272	0.304	3.664	0.627	0	23.52	0.648	124.16
0.88	6.86	1.05	1.72	0.339	0	5	0.308	65.9
4.389	26.22	1.539	1.026	0.148	0	99.18	1.425	264.48
5.95	36.455	2.198	0.251	0.046	0	12.56	0.597	7.85
5.031	44.772	3.51	1.755	0.351	0	19.5	0.819	9.75
4.25	44.509	0.632	0.442	0.122	0	15.8	1.896	603.56
11.34	47.53	1.47	2.59	1.26	9.8	92.4	2.562	561.4
6.678	39.676	1.82	0.938	0.133	0	9.8	1.96	1.4
6.215	54.24	2.938	7.345	1.579	33.9	64.41	1.819	505.11
6.667	57.517	3.842	9.492	1.53	29.38	83.62	3.175	588.73
3.771	25.893	1.755	13.842	1.973	0	9	2.128	197.55
7.6	39.744	1.76	2.352	0.496	52.8	19.2	2.544	11.2
2.432	10.754		3.686	0.806	22.42	83.22	0.684	166.82
6.678	39.676	2.38	0.938	0.133	0	9.8	1.96	1.4
18.648	108.617	21.016	14.06	2.094	0	16.28	3.374	725.2
3.268	19.076	1.216	1.634	0.366	0	34.58	1.03	231.42
4.085	21.264	0.903	1.862	0.47	0	59.34	1.428	205.97
2.828	18.032	1.484	5.544	0.664	0	17.08	0.826	82.32
2.072	18.844	1.288	4.816	2.027	0.28	29.4	0.717	77.84
0.96	6.232	1.208	0.336	0.046	0	0.8	0.213	0.32
1.476	14.67	0.756	0.504	0.103	0	1.98	0.268	
31.86	110.92	4.484	17.063	8.496	99.12	358.72	3.54	811.84
1.482	12.116	1.352	0.65	0.087	0	45.5	0.364	2.86
4.002	25.576	1.518	3.266	0.803	0	57.5	1.518	219.88
2.301	15.054	0.858	3.042	0.505	12.48	86.19	1.657	291.72

EvaluEat Code	Food Name	Amount	Wt (g)	Ener (kcal)
Protein Sources				
16104	Bacon, vegetarian, meatless	1 strip	5	15.5
16006	Beans, Baked, Plain or Vegetarian, canned	1 cup	254	236.22
16029	Beans, Kidney, mature seeds, canned	1 cup	256	207.36
16162	Beans, Soy, Tofu, Mori-Nu, silken, firm	1 slice	84	52.08
16051	Beans, White, mature seeds, canned	1 cup	262	306.54
16137	Beans, Hummus, Garbanzo or Chick Pea Spread, homemade	1 tbsp	15	26.55
13012	Beef, All Cuts, All Grades, lean (1/4"trim) cooked	3 oz	85	183.6
13306	Beef, Ground, lean, broiled, welldone	3 oz	85	238
13313	Beef, Ground, regular, broiled, welldone	3 oz	85	248.2
5009	Chicken, Broiler or Fryer, meat & skin, roasted	1 cup, chopped or diced	140	334.6
5012	Chicken, Broiler or Fryer, meat only, no skin, fried	1 cup, chopped or diced	140	306.6
5013	Chicken, Broiler or Fryer, meat only, no skin, roasted	1 cup, chopped or diced	140	266
43128	Chicken, meatless	1 cup	186	416.64
22904	Chili con carne w/beans, canned entree	1 serving	222	255.3
1143	Egg Substitute, liquid	1 cup	251	210.84
1128	Egg, Whole, fried	1 large	46	92.5
1129	Egg, Whole, hard-cooked	1 large	50	77.5
1131	Egg, Whole, poached	1 large	50	73.5
1132	Egg, Whole, scrambled	1 large	61	101.26
15087	Fish, Salmon, Sockeye w/bone, canned, drained	3 oz	85	130.05
15086	Fish, Salmon, Sockeye, baked or broiled (dry heat)	3 oz	85	183.6
15128	Fish, Tuna Salad	1 cup	205	383.35
15126	Fish, White Tuna, canned in H20, drained	3 oz	85	108.8
15124	Fish, White Tuna, canned in oil, drained	3 oz	85	158.1
7945	Frankfurter, beef, heated	1 serving	52	169.52
17002	Lamb, Domestic, Choice, Composite, lean&fat (1/4" trim) ckd	3 oz	85	249.9
7007	Lunch Meat, Bologna (Beef)	1 slice	28	87.08
7079	Lunch Meat, Turkey Breast Meat	1 slice	28	26.88
16097	Peanut Butter, chunky w/salt	2 tbsp	32	188.48
16098	Peanut Butter, smooth w/salt	2 tbsp	32	191.68
16390	Peanuts, All Types, dry roasted w/o salt	1 oz	28.35	165.848
16090	Peanuts, All Types, dry roasted w/salt	1 oz	28.35	165.848
22903	Pizza, Pepperoni, frozen	1 serving	146	400.04
22902	Pizza, Sausage & pepperoni, frozen	1 serving	146	385.44
10124	Pork Bacon, Cured, broiled, pan-fried, or roasted	1 slice, cooked	8	43.28
10188	Pork Composite (leg,loin/shoulder/sparerib) Fresh, lean&fat, ckd	3 oz	85	232.05
10220	Pork, Ground, Fresh, ckd	3 oz	85	252.45
7019	Sausage, Chorizo (Pork & Beef)	1 link (4" long)	60	273
7919	Sausage, Turkey, breakfast links, mild	1 serving	56	131.6
16107	Sausage, Vegetarian, Meatless	1 link	25	64.25

Prot (g)	Carb (g)	Fiber (g)	Fat (g)	Sat (g)	Chol (g)	Calc (mg)	Iron (mg)	Sodi (mg)
0.534	0.316	0.13	1.476	0.231	0	1.15	0.121	73.25
12.167	52.121	12.7	1.143	0.295	0	127	0.737	1008.38
13.312	38.093	8.96	0.794	0.115	0	69.12	3.149	888.32
5.796	2.016	0.084	2.268	0.341	0	26.88	0.865	30.24
19.021	57.483	12.576	0.76	0.194	0	191.26	7.834	13.1
0.729	3.018	0.6	0.312	0.168	0	7.35	25.95	
25.143	0	0	8.424	3.222	73.1	7.65	2.542	56.95
23.97	0	0	14.994	5.891	85.85	10.2	2.082	75.65
23.12	0	0	16.541	6.503	85.85	10.2	2.329	79.05
38.22	0	0	19.04	5.306	123.2	21	1.764	114.8
42.798	2.366	0.14	12.768	3.444	131.6	23.8	1.89	127.4
40.502	0	0	10.374	2.856	124.6	21	1.694	120.4
43.97	6.77	6.696	13.528	3.385	0	65.1	100.44	
20.18	24.487	8.214	8.147	2.109	24.42	66.6	3.308	1032.3
30.12	1.606	0	8.308	1.654	2.51	133.03	5.271	444.27
6.27	0.405	0		1.975	210.2	27.1	0.911	93.8
6.29	0.56	0	5.305	1.633	212	25	0.595	62
6.265	0.38	0	0.679	1.543	211	26.5	66.5	
6.765	1.342	0	7.448	2.244	214.72	43.31	0.732	170.8
17.399	0	0	6.214	1.397	37.4	203.15	0.901	457.3
23.214	0	0	9.325	1.629	73.95	5.95	0.468	56.1
32.882	19.29	0	18.983	3.165	26.65	34.85	2.05	824.1
20.077	0	0	2.525	0.673	35.7	11.9	0.825	320.45
22.551	0	0	6.868	1.088	26.35	3.4	0.553	336.6
6.001	1.96	0	15.319	5.947	29.12	6.24	0.811	600.08
20.842	0	0	17.799	7.506	82.45	14.45	1.598	61.2
2.876	1.114	0	7.893	3.118	15.68	8.68	0.308	302.4
2.044	3.822	0.56	0.378	0.118	3.36	3.08	0.33	47.04
8.022	6.749	2.112	15.904	3.066	0	16.96	0.653	150.4
7.99	5.894	1.888	16.73	3.209	0	15.04	0.602	160
6.713	6.098	2.268	14.079	1.954	0	15.309	0.641	1.701
6.713	6.098	2.268	14.079	1.954	0	15.309	0.641	230.486
16.191	36.208	2.336	21.112	7.066	33.58	0	2.613	878.92
15.768	36.179	2.336	19.695	6.336	30.66	191.26	2.774	854.1
2.963	0.114	0	3.342	1.099	8.8	0.88	0.115	184.8
23.434	0	0	14.603	5.287	77.35	21.25	0.935	52.7
21.837	0	0	17.655	6.562	79.9	18.7	1.097	62.05
14.46	1.116	0	22.962	8.628	52.8	4.8	0.954	741
8.635	0.874	0	10.13	4.002	33.6	17.92	0.599	327.6
4.633	2.46	0.7	4.54	0.732	0	15.75	0.93	222

EvaluEat Code	Food Name	Amount	Wt (g)	Ener (kcal)
15151	Shellfish, Shrimp, boiled/steamed (moist heat)	4 large	22	21.78
15150	Shellfish, Shrimp, breaded & fried	4 large	30	72.6
43133	Soyburger	1 cup	186	332.94
42130	Turkey bacon, cooked	1 ounce	28.34	108.259
5220	Turkey, Fryer/Roaster, Breast, no skin, roasted	1 unit (yield from 1 lb) ready-to-cook turkey	87	117.45
5208	Turkey, Fryer/Roaster, Dark Meat w/skin, roasted	1 unit (yield from 1 lb ready-to-cook turkey)	106	192.92
5206	Turkey, Fryer/Roaster, Light Meat w/skin, roasted	1 unit (yield from 1 lb ready-to-cook turkey)	123	201.72
5306	Turkey, Ground, cooked	1 patty (4 oz, raw)	82	192.7
17089	Veal, Composite, lean & fat, cooked	3 oz	85	196.35
43137	Vegetarian meatloaf or patties	1 cup	186	366.42
43136	Vegetarian stew	1 cup	186	228.78

Dairy

EvaluEat Code	Food Name	Amount	Wt (g)	Ener (kcal)
43276	Cheese spread, cream cheese base	1 cup	186	548.7
1009	Cheese, Cheddar	1 cup, shredded	113	455.39
1012	Cheese, Cottage, Creamed, large or small curd	4 oz	113	116.39
1015	Cheese, Cottage, Lowfat, 2% fat	4 oz	113	101.7
1014	Cheese, Cottage, Nonfat, Uncreamed, Dry, large or small curd	4 oz	113	96.05
1017	Cheese, Cream	1 tbsp	14.5	50.605
1186	Cheese, Cream, fat free	1 ounce	28.34	27.206
1168	Cheese, Cheddar or Colby, low fat	1 cup, shredded	113	195.49
1028	Cheese, Mozzarella, Part Skim Milk	1 oz	28.35	72.009
1026	Cheese, Mozzarella, Whole Milk	1 oz	28.35	85.05
1032	Cheese, Parmesan, grated	1 tbsp	5	21.55
42205	Cheese, pasteurized process, cheddar or american, fat-free	1 cup	186	275.28
1037	Cheese, Ricotta, Part Skim Milk	1 cup	246	339.48
1049	Cream, Half and Half	1 tbsp	15	19.5
1053	Cream, Heavy Whipping	1 cup, whipped	120	414
42185	Frozen yogurts, chocolate, nonfat milk, with low calorie sweetener	1 cup	186	199.02
42187	Frozen yogurts, flavors other than chocolate	1 cup	186	236.22
1082	Milk, Lowfat, 1% fat w/added vitamin A	1 cup	244	102.48
1104	Milk, Lowfat, 1% fat, Chocolate	1 cup	250	157.5
1085	Milk, Nonfat/Fat Free, Skim w/added Vit A	1 cup	245	83.3
16120	Milk, Soy, fluid	1 cup	245	120.05
1077	Milk, Whole, 3.25% fat	1 cup	244	146.4
1102	Milk, Whole, Chocolate	1 cup	250	207.5
1180	Sour cream, fat free	1 ounce	28.34	20.972
1179	Sour cream, light	1 ounce	28.34	38.542
43261	Yogurt, fruit variety, nonfat	1 cup	186	174.84
1121	Yogurt, Lowfat w/fruit, 10g protein/8 oz	1 cup (8 fl oz)	245	249.9
1117	Yogurt, Lowfat, Plain, 12g protein/8 oz	1 cup (8 fl oz)	245	154.35
1116	Yogurt, Whole Milk, Plain, 8g protein/8 oz	1 cup (8 fl oz)	245	149.45

Prot (g)	Carb (g)	Fiber (g)	Fat (g)	Sat (g)	Chol (g)	Calc (mg)	Iron (mg)	Sodi (mg)
4.6	0	0	0.238	0.064	42.9	8.58	0.68	49.28
6.417	3.441	0.12	3.684	0.626	53.1	20.1	0.378	103.2
33.313	24.924	8.556	11.104	1.337	0	53.94	3.906	1023
8.389	0.879	0	7.907	2.351	27.773	2.551	0.598	647.569
26.152	0	0	0.644	0.209	72.21	10.44	1.331	45.24
29.351	0	0	7.484	2.247	124.02	28.62	2.47	80.56
35.387	0	0	5.633	1.538	116.85	22.14	1.98	70.11
22.435	0	0	10.783	2.78	83.64	20.5	1.583	87.74
25.585	0	0	9.682	3.638	96.9	18.7	0.978	73.95
39.06	14.88	8.556	16.74	2.65	0	53.94	3.906	1023
31.62	13.02	2.046	5.58	0.883	0	57.66	2.418	744
13.206	6.51	0	53.196	33.517	167.4	132.06	2.102	1251.78
28.137	1.446	0	37.448	23.834	118.65	814.73	0.768	701.73
14.114	3.028	0	5.096	3.224	16.95	67.8	0.158	457.65
15.526	4.102	0	2.181	1.38	9.04	77.97	0.181	458.78
19.515	2.091	0	0.475	0.308	7.91	36.16	0.26	14.69
1.095	0.386	0	5.056	3.185	15.95	11.6	0.174	42.92
4.084	1.644	0	0.385	0.255	2.267	52.429	0.051	154.453
27.516	2.158	0	0.251	4.906	23.73	468.95	74.58	
6.878	0.785	0	4.513	2.867	18.144	221.697	0.062	175.487
6.285	0.621	0	6.336	3.729	22.397	143.168	0.125	177.755
1.923	0.203	0	1.431	0.865	4.4	55.45	0.045	76.45
41.85	24.924	0	1.488	0.937	20.46	1281.54	0.521	2842.08
28.019	12.644	0	19.459	12.12	76.26	669.12	1.082	307.5
0.444	0.645	0	1.725	1.074	5.55	15.75	0.011	6.15
2.46	3.348	0	1.649	27.638	164.4	78	90	
8.184	36.642	3.72	1.488	0.939	7.44	295.74	0.074	150.66
5.58	40.176	0	6.696	4.326	24.18	186	0.856	117.18
8.223	12.176	0	2.367	1.545	12.2	263.52	0.854	122
8.1	26.1	1.25	2.5	1.54	7.5	287.5	0.6	152.5
8.257	12.152	0	0.196	0.287	4.9	222.95	1.225	107.8
9.188	11.368	3.185	5.096	0.524	0	9.8	1.421	29.4
7.857	11.029	0	7.93	4.551	24.4	246.44	0.073	104.92
7.925	25.85	2	8.475	5.26	30	280	0.6	150
0.879	4.421	0	0	0	2.551	35.425	0	39.959
0.992	2.012	0	3.004	1.87	9.919	39.959	0.02	20.121
8.184	35.34	0	0.372	0.221	3.72	282.72	0.13	107.88
10.707	46.673	0	2.646	1.708	9.8	372.4	0.171	142.1
12.863	17.248	0	3.797	2.45	14.7	448.35	0.196	171.5
8.502	11.417	0	7.963	5.135	31.85	296.45	0.123	112.7

EvaluEat Code	Food Name	Amount	Wt (g)	Ener (kcal)
Fruits				
9103	Fruit Salad (peach, pineapple, pear, apricot & cherry) canned in juice	1 cup	249	124.5
9003	Fruit, Apple w/skin, raw	1 large (3-1/4" dia) (approx 2 per lb)	212	110.24
9007	Fruit, Apple, slices, sweetened, canned, drained	1 cup slices	204	136.68
9402	Fruit, Applesauce, canned, sweetened w/added Vit C	1 cup	255	193.8
9401	Fruit, Applesauce, canned, unsweetened w/ added Vit C	1 cup	244	104.92
9021	Fruit, Apricot, raw	1 apricot	35	16.8
9038	Fruit, Avocado, California, peeled, raw	1 fruit without skin and seeds	173	288.91
9040	Fruit, Banana, peeled, raw, mashed/sliced	1 medium (7" to 7-7/8" long)	118	105.02
9050	Fruit, Blueberries, raw	1 cup	145	82.65
9070	Fruit, Cherries, Sweet, raw	1 cup, with pits, yields	117	73.71
9087	Fruit, Dates, Domestic, Natural, dried	1 cup, pitted, chopped	178	501.96
9089	Fruit, Figs, raw	1 large (2-1/2" dia)	64	47.36
9111	Fruit, Grapefruit, Red, White or Pink, peeled, raw	.5 medium (approx 4" dia)	128	40.96
9131	Fruit, Grapes, American type (slip skin) raw	1 cup	92	61.64
9148	Fruit, Kiwifruit (Chinese Gooseberry) peeled, raw	1 fruit without skin, medium	76	46.36
9176	Fruit, Mango, peeled, raw	1 cup, sliced	165	107.25
9184	Fruit, Melon, Honeydew, peeled, wedges, raw	1 wedge (1/8 of 6" to 7" dia melon)	160	57.6
9191	Fruit, Nectarine, raw	1 fruit (2-1/2" dia)	136	59.84
9200	Fruit, Orange, All Varieties, peeled, raw	1 fruit (2-5/8" dia)	131	61.57
9226	Fruit, Papayas, peeled, cubed/mashed, raw	1 medium (5-1/8" long x 3" dia)	304	118.56
9236	Fruit, Peach, peeled, raw	1 medium (2-1/2" dia) (approx 4 per lb)	98	38.22
9252	Fruit, Pear, raw	1 pear, medium (approx 2-1/2 per lb)	166	96.28
9279	Fruit, Plum, raw	1 fruit (2-1/8" dia)	66	30.36
9291	Fruit, Prunes, dried	1 prune	8.4	20.16
9298	Fruit, Raisins, seedless	1 cup (not packed)	145	433.55
9302	Fruit, Raspberries, raw	1 cup	123	63.96
9316	Fruit, Strawberries, halves/slices, raw	1 cup, halves	152	48.64
9326	Fruit, Watermelon, balls, raw	1 cup, balls	154	46.2
Vegetables				
11358	Potatoes, red, flesh and skin, baked	1 potato, large (3" to 4-1/4" dia)	299	266.11
11356	Potatoes, Russet, flesh and skin, baked	1 potato, large	299	290.03
11702	Vege, Artichokes (Globe or French) boiled w/ salt, drained	1 artichoke, medium	120	60
11705	Vege, Asparagus, boiled w/salt, drained	4 spears (1/2" base)	60	13.2
11723	Vege, Beans, Snap, Green, boiled w/salt, drained	1 cup	125	43.75
11734	Vege, Beets, boiled w/salt, drained	.5 cup slices	85	37.4

Prot (g)	Carb (g)	Fiber (g)	Fat (g)	Sat (g)	Chol (g)	Calc (mg)	Iron (mg)	Sodi (mg)
1.27	32.494	2.49	0.075	0.01	0	27.39	0.623	12.45
0.551	29.277	5.088	0.36	0.059	0	12.72	0.254	2.12
0.367	34.068	3.468	1	0.163	0	8.16	0.469	6.12
0.459	50.771	3.06	0.459	0.076	0	10.2	0.892	71.4
0.415	27.548	2.928	0.122	0.02	0	7.32	0.293	4.88
0.49	3.892	0.7	0.136	0.009	0	4.55	0.136	0.35
3.391	14.947	11.764	26.659	3.678	0	22.49	1.055	13.84
1.286	26.951	3.068	0.389	0.132	0	5.9	0.307	1.18
1.073	21.01	3.48	0.479	0.041	0	8.7	0.406	1.45
1.24	18.732	2.457	0.234	0.044	0	15.21	0.421	0
4.361	133.553	14.24	0.694	0.057	0	69.42	1.816	3.56
0.48	12.275	1.856	0.192	0.038	0	22.4	0.237	0.64
0.806	10.342	1.408	0.128	0.018	0	15.36	0.115	0
0.58	15.778	0.828	0.322	0.105	0	12.88	0.267	1.84
0.866	11.142	2.28	0.395	0.022	0	25.84	0.236	2.28
0.841	28.05	2.97	0.446	0.109	0	16.5	0.214	3.3
0.864	14.544	1.28	0.224	0.061	0	9.6	0.272	28.8
1.442	14.348	2.312	0.435	0.034	0	8.16	0.381	0
1.231	15.392	3.144	0.157	0.02	0	52.4	0.131	0
1.854	29.822	5.472	0.426	0.131	0	72.96	0.304	9.12
0.892	9.349	1.47	0.245	0.019	0	5.88	0.245	0
0.631	25.664	5.146	0.199	0.01	0	14.94	0.282	1.66
0.462	7.537	0.924	0.185	0.011	0	3.96	0.112	0
0.183	5.366	0.596	0.032	0.007	0	3.612	0.078	0.168
4.451	114.811	5.365	0.667	0.084	0	72.5	2.726	15.95
1.476	14.686	7.995	0.799	0.023	0	30.75	0.849	1.23
1.018	11.674	3.04	0.456	0.023	0	24.32	0.638	1.52
0.939	11.627	0.616	0.231	0.025	0	10.78	0.37	1.54
6.877	58.574	5.382	0.449	0.078	0	26.91	2.093	23.92
7.864	64.106	6.877	0.389		0	53.82	3.199	23.92
4.176	13.416	6.48	0.192	0.044	0	54	1.548	397.2
1.44	2.466	1.2	0.132	0.043	0	13.8	0.546	144
2.362	9.863	4	0.35	0.08	0	57.5	1.6	298.75
1.428	8.466	1.7	0.153	0.024	0	13.6	0.672	242.25

EvaluEat Code	Food Name	Amount	Wt (g)	Ener (kcal)
11741	Vege, Broccoli Stalks, raw	1 stalk	114	31.92
11742	Vege, Broccoli, boiled w/salt, chopped, drained	.5 cup, chopped	78	21.84
11745	Vege, Brussels Sprouts, boiled w/salt, drained	.5 cup	78	31.98
11109	Vege, Cabbage Heads, raw	1 cup, chopped	89	21.36
11960	Vege, Carrots, Baby, raw	1 medium	10	3.5
11757	Vege, Carrots, boiled w/salt, drained	.5 cup slices	78	27.3
11761	Vege, Cauliflower, boiled w/salt, drained	.5 cup (1" pieces)	62	14.26
11143	Vege, Celery, raw	1 cup, diced	120	16.8
11765	Vege, Chard, Swiss, boiled w/salt, drained	1 cup, chopped	175	35
11768	Vege, Collards, boiled w/salt, drained	1 cup, chopped	190	49.4
11900	Vege, Corn, White, Sweet, ears, raw	1 ear, large	143	122.98
11176	Vege, Corn, Yellow, Sweet, canned, vacuum/ regular pack	.5 cup	105	82.95
11205	Vege, Cucumber, raw	.5 cup slices	52	7.8
11783	Vege, Eggplant (Brinjal) boiled w/salt, drained	1 cup (1" cubes)	99	34.65
11260	Vege, Fungi, Mushrooms, slices, raw	1 medium	18	3.96
11790	Vege, Kale, boiled w/salt, drained	1 cup, chopped	130	36.4
11251	Vege, Lettuce, Cos/Romaine, raw	1 inner leaf	10	1.7
11252	Vege, Lettuce, Iceberg, head, raw	1 head, medium	539	53.9
11300	Vege, Peas w/edible pod-Snow/Sugar, raw	1 cup, chopped	98	41.16
11811	Vege, Peas, Green, boiled w/salt, drained	1 cup	160	134.4
11308	Vege, Peas, Green, canned, regular pack, drained	1 cup	170	117.3
11979	Vege, Pepper, Jalapeno, raw	1 cup, sliced	90	27
11333	Vege, Pepper, Sweet, Green, chopped/sliced, raw	1 medium	119	23.8
11821	Vege, Pepper, Sweet, Red, raw	1 medium	119	30.94
11833	Vege, Potato, boiled w/o skin & w/salt	1 medium	167	143.62
11838	Vege, Potato, French Fries, frozen, oven heated, w/salt	10 strips	50	100
11854	Vege, Spinach, boiled w/salt, drained	1 cup	180	41.4
11457	Vege, Spinach, raw	1 cup	30	6.9
11857	Vege, Squash, Summer, All Varieties, boiled w/salt, drained	1 cup slices	180	36
11863	Vege, Squash, Winter, All Varieties, baked w/salt	1 cup, cubes	205	79.95
11875	Vege, Sweet Potato, baked in skin w/salt	1 medium (2" dia, 5" long, raw)	114	102.6
11529	Vege, Tomato, Red, ripe, whole, raw	1 cup, chopped or sliced	180	32.4
11897	Vege, Yam, boiled or baked w/salt	1 cup, cubes	136	157.76
11894	Vegetables, Mixed, frozen, boiled w/salt, drained	.5 cup	91	53.69

Fast Food

Breakfast Items

21023	Fast Food, French Toast w/butter	2 slices	135	356.4
21025	Fast Food, Pancakes w/butter & syrup	2 cakes	232	519.68
21026	Fast Food, Potatoes, Hash Brown	.5 cup	72	151.2
21002	Fast Food, Sandwich, Biscuit w/egg	1 biscuit	136	372.64
21003	Fast Food, Sandwich, Biscuit w/egg & bacon	1 biscuit	150	457.5
21004	Fast Food, Sandwich, Biscuit w/egg & ham	1 biscuit	192	441.6
21005	Fast Food, Sandwich, Biscuit w/egg & sausage	1 biscuit	180	581.4
21007	Fast Food, Sandwich, Biscuit w/egg, cheese & bacon	1 biscuit	144	476.64

Prot (g)	Carb (g)	Fiber (g)	Fat (g)	Sat (g)	Chol (g)	Calc (mg)	Iron (mg)	Sodi (mg)
3.397	5.974		0.399	0.062	0	54.72	1.003	30.78
2.324	3.947	2.574	0.273	0.042	0	31.2	0.523	204.36
1.989	6.763	2.028	0.398	0.082	0	28.08	0.936	200.46
1.282	4.966	2.047	0.107	0.014	0	41.83	0.525	16.02
0.064	0.824	0.18	0.013	0.002	0	3.2	0.089	7.8
0.593	6.412	2.34	0.14	0.023	0	23.4	0.265	235.56
1.141	2.548	1.674	0.279	0.043	0	9.92	0.205	150.04
0.828	3.564	1.92	0.204	0.052	0	48	0.24	96
3.29	7.227	3.675	0.14		0	101.5	3.955	726.25
4.009	9.329	5.32	0.684	0.089	0	266	2.204	478.8
4.605	27.199	3.861	1.687	0.26	0	2.86	0.744	21.45
2.53	20.412	2.1	0.525	0.081	0	5.25	0.441	285.6
0.338	1.888	0.26	0.057	0.018	0	8.32	0.146	1.04
0.822	8.643	2.475	0.228	0.044	0	5.94	0.248	236.61
0.56	0.583	0.216	0.061	0.008	0	0.54	0.094	0.72
2.47	7.319	2.6	0.52	0.068	0	93.6	1.17	336.7
0.123	0.329	0.21	0.03	0.004	0	3.3	0.097	0.8
4.366	11.265	5.39	0.593	0.075	0	107.8	1.886	48.51
2.744	7.399	2.548	0.196	0.038	0	42.14	2.038	3.92
8.576	25.024	8.8	0.352	0.062	0	43.2	2.464	382.4
7.514	21.386	6.97	0.595	0.105	0	34	1.615	428.4
1.215	5.319	2.52	0.558	0.056	0	9	0.63	0.9
1.023	5.522	2.023	0.202	0.069	0	11.9	0.405	3.57
1.178	7.176	2.38	0.357	0.07	0	8.33	0.512	2.38
2.856	33.417	3.34	0.167	0.043	0	13.36	0.518	402.47
1.585	15.595	1.6	3.78	0.631	0	4	0.62	133
5.346	6.75	4.32	0.468	0.076	0	244.8	6.426	550.8
0.858	1.089	0.66	0.117	0.019	0	29.7	0.813	23.7
1.638	7.758	2.52	0.558	0.115	0	48.6	0.648	426.6
1.824	17.938	5.74	1.291	0.266	0	28.7	0.677	485.85
2.291	23.609	3.762	0.171	0.039	0	43.32	0.787	280.44
1.584	7.056	2.16	0.36	0.081	0	18	0.486	9
2.026	37.509	5.304	0.19	0.039	0	19.04	0.707	331.84
2.603	11.912	4.004	0.137	0.028	0	22.75	0.746	246.61
10.341	36.045		18.765	7.749	116.1	72.9	1.89	513
8.259	90.898		13.99	5.851	58	127.6	2.622	1104.32
1.944	16.15		9.216	4.324	9.36	7.2	0.482	290.16
11.601	31.906	0.816	22.073	4.729	244.8	81.6	2.897	890.8
16.995	28.59	0.75	31.095	7.95	352.5	189	3.735	999
20.429	30.317	0.768	27.034	5.914	299.52	220.8	4.55	1382.4
19.152	41.148	0.9	38.7	14.976	302.4	154.8	3.96	1141.2
16.258	33.422		31.392	11.398	260.64	164.16	2.549	1260

EvaluEat Code	Food Name	Amount	Wt (g)	Ener (kcal)
Chicken				
21035	Fast Food, Chicken, breaded, fried, dark meat (drumstick or thigh)	2 pieces	148	430.68
21036	Fast Food, Chicken, breaded, fried, light meat (breast or wing)	2 pieces	163	493.89
21102	Fast Food, Sandwich, Chicken Filet, plain	1 sandwich	182	515.06
Burgers				
21098	Fast Food, Sandwich, Cheeseburger, large, one meat patty w/condiments & veges	1 sandwich	219	562.83
21109	Fast Food, Sandwich, Hamburger, one patty w/condiments & veges	1 sandwich	110	279.4
21107	Fast Food, Sandwich, Hamburger, plain	1 sandwich	90	274.5
Mexican				
21061	Fast Food, Burrito w/beans & cheese	2 pieces	186	377.58
21066	Fast Food, Burrito w/beef	2 pieces	220	523.6
21082	Fast Food, Taco	1 large	263	568.08
Sides/Beverages/Other				
21118	Fast Food, Hot Dog, plain	1 sandwich	98	242.06
21033	Fast Food, Ice Cream Sundae, hot fudge	1 sundae	158	284.4
14346	Fast Food, Milk Beverage, Chocolate Shake/McDonald's	1 medium shake (16 fl oz)	333	422.91
14347	Fast Food, Shake, Vanilla/McDonald's	1 medium shake (16 fl oz)	333	369.63
21130	Fast Food, Onion Rings, breaded, fried	1 portion (8-9 onion rings)	83	275.56
21049	Fast Food, Pizza w/cheese	1 slice	63	140.49
21050	Fast Food, Pizza w/cheese, meat & veges	1 slice	79	184.07
21138	Fast Food, Potato, French fried w/vegetable oil	1 large	169	577.98
21105	Fast Food, Sandwich, Fish w/tartar sauce	1 sandwich	158	431.34
Beverages				
14006	Beverage, Alcoholic, Beer, Light	1 can or bottle (12 fl oz)	354	99.12
14003	Beverage, Alcoholic, Beer, Regular	1 can	356	117.48
14049	Beverage, Alcoholic, Distilled Spirits, Gin, Vodka, Rum, Whiskey	1 jigger 1.5 fl oz	42	110.46
14084	Beverage, Alcoholic, Wine (all table)	1 glass 3.5 fl oz	103	79.31
14209	Beverage, Coffee, Brewed	1 cup (8 fl oz)	237	9.48
14400	Beverage, Cola w/caffeine	1 can 12 fl oz	370	155.4
14177	Beverage Mix, Chocolate Flavor, dry mix, prep w/milk	1 cup (8 fl oz)	266	226.1
14351	Beverage Mix, Strawberry Flavor, dry, prep w/milk	1 cup (8 fl oz)	266	234.08
14182	Beverage, Chocolate Syrup w/o added nutrients, prep w/milk	1 cup (8 fl oz)	282	253.8
14194	Beverage, Cocoa Mix, dry, w/o added nutrients, prep w/H_2O	1 oz packet with 6 fl oz water	206	113.3
14136	Beverage, Soft Drink, Ginger Ale	1 can or bottle (16 fl oz)	488	165.92
14145	Beverage, Soft Drink, Lemon-Lime	1 can or bottle (16 fl oz)	491	196.4
14153	Beverage, Soft Drink, Pepper type	1 can or bottle (16 fl oz)	491	201.31

Prot (g)	Carb (g)	Fiber (g)	Fat (g)	Sat (g)	Chol (g)	Calc (mg)	Iron (mg)	Sodi (mg)
30.074	15.703		26.699	7.049	165.76	35.52	1.598	754.8
35.713	19.576		29.519	7.844	148.33	60.31	1.483	974.74
24.115	38.693		29.448	8.527	60.06	60.06	4.677	957.32
28.185	38.391		32.938	15.039	87.6	205.86	4.665	1108.14
12.914	27.291		13.475	4.131	26.4	62.7	2.629	503.8
12.321	30.51		11.817	4.141	35.1	63	2.403	387
15.066	54.963		11.699	6.849	27.9	213.9	2.269	1166.22
26.598	58.52		20.812	10.459	63.8	83.6	6.094	1491.6
31.77	41.107		31.613	17.484	86.79	339.27	3.708	1233.47
10.388	18.032		14.543	5.109	44.1	23.52	2.313	670.32
5.641	47.669	0	8.627	5.023	20.54	206.98	0.585	181.7
11.322	68.265	6.327	12.321	7.702	43.29	376.29	1.032	323.01
11.655	59.607	0.333	9.99	6.187	36.63	406.26	0.3	273.06
3.702	31.324		15.513	6.953	14.11	73.04	0.847	429.94
7.68	20.5		3.213	1.54	9.45	116.55	0.58	335.79
13.011	21.291		5.364	1.535	20.54	101.12	1.533	382.36
7.267	67.279	5.915	31.147	6.507	0	23.66	1.318	334.62
16.938	41.017		22.768	5.235	55.3	83.74	2.607	614.62
0.708	4.602	0	0	0	0	17.7	0.142	10.62
1.068	5.732	0.356	0.214	0	0	17.8	0.071	14.24
0	0	0	0	0	0	0	0	0.84
0.206	3.296	0	0	0	0	8.24	0.36	6.18
0.332	0	0	1.801	0	0	2.37	0.024	2.37
0.185	39.775	0	0	0	0	11.1	0.074	14.8
8.592	31.681	1.064	0.495	4.948	23.94	252.7	457.52	
7.98	32.718	0	0.303	5.081	31.92	292.6	369.74	
8.657	36.04	0.846	0.485	4.74	25.38	250.98	408.9	
1.669	23.978	1.03	0.035	0.672	2.06	45.32	201.88	
0	42.798	0	0	0	0	14.64	0.878	34.16
0	51.064	0	0	0	0	9.82	0.344	54.01
0	51.064	0	0.491	0.344	0	14.73	0.196	49.1

EvaluEat Code	Food Name	Amount	Wt (g)	Ener (kcal)
14355	Beverage, Tea, Brewed	1 cup (8 fl oz)	237	2.37
9206	Fruit Juice, Orange, fresh	1 cup	248	111.6
9215	Fruit Juice, Orange, frozen concentrate, unsweetened, prep	1 cup	249	112.05
9016	Fruit Juice, Apple, canned or bottled, unsweetened w/o added Vit C	1 cup	248	116.56
9018	Fruit Juice, Apple, frozen concentrate, unsweetened w/o added Vit C, prep	1 cup	239	112.33
Fats/Sweets/Other				
16124	Bean Sauce, Soy (Tamari)	1 tsp	6	3.6
1001	Butter, Regular (with salt)	1 tbsp	14.2	101.814
1002	Butter, Whipped (with salt)	1 tbsp	9.4	67.398
43031	Candies, chocolate covered, caramel with nuts	1 cup	186	874.2
19120	Candy, Milk Chocolate	1 bar 1.55 oz	44	235.4
19126	Candy, Peanuts, milk chocolate coated	10 pieces	40	207.6
19127	Candy, Raisins, milk chocolate coated	10 pieces	10	39
19434	Cheese puffs and twists, corn based, low fat	1 oz	28.35	122.472
18154	Cookie, Brownies, homemade	1 brownie (2" square)	24	111.84
18378	Cookie, Chocolate Chip, homemade w/butter	1 cookie, medium (2-1/4" dia)	16	78.08
18184	Cookie, Oatmeal, homemade w/raisins	1 cookie (2-5/8" dia)	15	65.25
1054	Cream, Whipped Cream Topping, Pressurized	1 tbsp	3	7.71
19270	Ice Cream, Chocolate	.5 cup (4 fl oz)	66	142.56
19271	Ice Cream, Strawberry	.5 cup (4 fl oz)	66	126.72
19095	Ice Cream, Vanilla	1 tsp	4.7	33.793
4067	Margarine, Hard, Corn, Soybean-Hydrogenated & Cottonseed-Hydrogenated w/salt	1 tsp	4.7	33.793
4611	Margarine, regular, tub, composite, 80% fat, with salt	1 tbsp	12.8	91.648
1110	Milk Shake, Thick, Chocolate	1 container (10.6 oz)	300	357
1111	Milk Shake, Thick, Vanilla	1 container (11 oz)	313	350.56
4053	Oil, Vegetable/Salad/Cooking, Olive	1 tbsp	13.5	119.34
18239	Pastry, Croissant, Butter	1 croissant, mini	28	113.68
18301	Pie, Apple, enriched, commercially prep	1 piece (1/8 of 9" dia)	125	296.25
4017	Salad Dressing, 1000 Island, regular, w/salt	1 tbsp	16	59.2
4635	Salad dressing, 1000 Island dressing, fat-free	1 tbsp	14.6	19.272
4636	Salad dressing, Italian dressing, fat-free	1 tbsp	14.6	6.862
4114	Salad Dressing, Italian, regular w/salt	1 tbsp	14.7	42.777
4026	Salad Dressing, Mayonnaise, regular, Safflower/Soybean Oil, w/salt	1 tbsp	13.8	98.946
4012	Salad dressing, Miracle Whip Light Dressing/Kraft	1 tbsp	16	36.96
4638	Salad dressing, ranch dressing, fat-free	1 tbsp	14.6	17.374
4135	Salad Dressing, Vinegar & Oil, homemade	1 tbsp	16	71.84
6930	Sauce, cheese, ready-to-eat	.25 cup	63	109.62
6931	Sauce, Pasta, Spaghetti/Marinara	1 cup	250	142.5
6164	Sauce, Salsa	1 cup	259	72.52
19003	Snack, Corn Chips, Plain	1 oz	28.35	152.807

Prot (g)	Carb (g)	Fiber (g)	Fat (g)	Sat (g)	Chol (g)	Calc (mg)	Iron (mg)	Sodi (mg)
0	0.711	0	0	0.005	0	0	0.047	7.11
1.736	25.792	0.496	0.099	0.06	0	27.28	0.496	2.48
1.693	26.842	0.498	0.03	0.017	0	22.41	0.249	2.49
0.149	28.966	0.248	0.082	0.002	0	18.96	225.15	7.44
0.335	27.581	0.239	0.074	0.047	0	17.36	295.12	16.73
0.631	0.334	0.048	0.003	0.001	0	1.2	12.72	
0.121	0.009	0	11.518	5.799	30.53	3.408	0.003	81.792
0.08	0.006	0	7.624	4.746	20.586	2.256	0.015	77.738
17.67	112.846	7.998	39.06	8.662	0	145.08	3.162	44.64
3.366	26.136	1.496	13.05	6.271	10.12	83.16	1.034	34.76
5.24	19.76	1.88	13.4	5.84	3.6	41.6	0.524	16.4
0.41	6.83	0.42	1.48	0.88	0.3	8.6	0.171	3.6
2.41	20.511	3.033	3.43	0.595	0.284	101.21	0.363	364.298
1.488	12.048		6.984	1.757	17.52	13.68	0.442	82.32
0.912	9.312		4.544	2.251	11.2	6.08	0.397	54.56
0.975	10.26		2.43	0.485	4.95	15	0.398	80.7
0.096	0.375	0	0.667	0.415	2.28	3.03	0.002	3.9
2.508	18.612	0.792	7.26	4.488	22.44	71.94	0.614	50.16
2.112	18.216	0.594	5.544	3.425	19.14	79.2	0.139	39.6
0.042	0.042	0	3.783	0.705	0	1.41	0	
0.042	0.042	0	3.783	0.705	0	1.41	0	44.321
0.102	0.077	0	10.291	1.66	0	3.328	0	138.112
9.15	63.45	0.9	8.1	5.043	33	396	0.93	333
12.082	55.558	0	9.484	5.903	37.56	456.98	0.313	297.35
0	0	0	13.5	1.816	0	0.135	0.089	0.405
2.296	12.824	0.728	5.88	3.265	18.76	10.36	0.568	208.32
2.375	42.5	2	13.75	4.746	0	13.75	0.563	332.5
0.174	2.342	0.128	5.61	0.815	4.16	2.72	0.189	138.08
0.08	4.273	0.482	0.212	0.029	0.73	1.606	0.041	106.434
0.142	1.278	0.088	0.127	0.043	0.292	4.38	0.058	164.834
0.056	1.533	0	4.17	0.658	0	1.029	0.093	243.138
0.152	0.373	0	10.957	1.187	8.142	2.484	0.069	78.384
0.096	2.304	0.016	2.976	0.464	4.16	0.8	0.027	131.36
0.036	3.87	0.015	0.28	0.075	1.022	7.3	0.153	110.23
0	0.4	0	8.016	1.456	0	0	0	0.16
4.227	4.303	0.315	8.373	3.786	18.27	115.92	0.132	521.64
3.55	20.55	4	5.15	0.737	0	55	1.8	1030
3.289	16.162	4.144	0.622	0.078	0	77.7	2.512	1124.06
1.871	16.131	1.389	9.469	1.29	0	36.005	0.374	178.605

EvaluEat Code	Food Name	Amount	Wt (g)	Ener (kcal)
19411	Snack, Potato Chips, Plain, salted	1 oz	28.35	151.956
19047	Snack, Pretzel, Hard, Plain, salted	10 twists	60	228.6
19056	Snack, Tortilla Chips, Plain	1 oz	28.35	142.034
6008	Soup, Beef Broth or Bouillon, canned	1 cup	240	16.8
6413	Soup, Chicken Broth, canned, made w/H2O	1 cup	240	38.4
6583	Soup, ramen noodle, any flavor, dehydrated, dry	1 container, individual	64	289.92
19296	Sweet, Honey, strained/extracted	1 tbsp	21	63.84
19297	Sweet, Jams & Preserves	1 tbsp	20	55.6
19335	Sweet, Sugar, granulated, white	1 tsp	4.2	16.254
19129	Sweet, Syrup, pancake	1 tbsp	20	46.8
1073	Whipped Dessert Topping, Nondairy, semi solid, frozen	1 tbsp	4	12.72

Prot (g)	Carb (g)	Fiber (g)	Fat (g)	Sat (g)	Chol (g)	Calc (mg)	Iron (mg)	Sodi (mg)
1.985	14.997	1.276	9.809	3.107	0	6.804	0.462	168.399
5.46	47.52	1.92	2.1	0.45	0	21.6	2.592	1029
1.985	17.832	1.843	7.428	1.423	0	43.659	0.431	149.688
2.736	0.096	0	0.528	0.264	0	14.4	0.408	782.4
4.848	0.912	0	1.368	0.384	0	9.6	0.504	763.2
5.952	41.92	1.536	1.667	4.883	0	10.24	76.8	
0.063	17.304	0.042	0	0	0	1.26	0.088	0.84
0.074	13.772	0.22	0.014	0.002	0	4	0.098	6.4
0	4.199	0	0	0	0	0.042	0	0
0	12.294	0.14	0	0	0	0.6	0.006	16.4
0.05	0.922	0	1.012	0.871	0	0.24	0.005	1

Nutritional Content of Fast Foods

	Serving Size	Gram Weight	Calories (kcals)	Protein (g)	Carbohydrate (g)	Total Fat (g)	Saturated Fat (g)	% kcal from Fat	Cholesterol (mg)	Sodium (mg)	Fiber (g)	Sugars (g)	Calcium (mg)	Iron (mg)	Vitamin A (IU)	Vitamin C (mg)
KFC – Sides																
Barbecue Baked Beans	5.5 Oz	156	190	6	33	3	1	14.75	5	760	6	13	80	1.80	400	
Cole Slaw	5 Oz	142	232	2	26	13.50	2	52.03	8	284	3	20	30		450	34.20
Potato Salad	5.6 Oz	160	230	4	23	14	2	53.85	15	540	3	9	20	2.70	500	
Potato Wedges	4.8 Oz	135	280	5	28	13	4	46.99	5	750	5	1	20	1.80		1.20
Potato, Mashed w/Gravy	4.8 Oz	136	120	1	17	6	1	42.86	1	440	2	0		0.36		
KFC – Chicken																
Wing, Honey Barbecue	6 Pieces	189	607	33	33	38	10	56.44	193	1145	1	18	40	1.44	400	4.80
Wing, Hot	6 Pieces	135	471	27	18	33	8	62.26	150	1230	2	0	40	1.44		
Breast, Extra Crispy	1 Breast	168	470	39	17	28	8	52.94	160	874	1	0	20	1.08		
Breast, Original Recipe	1 Breast	153	400	29	16	24	6	54.55	135	1116	1	0	40	1.08		
Drumstick, Extra Crispy	1 Drumstk	67	195	15	7	12	3	55.10	77	375	1	0		0.72		
Drumstick, Original Recipe	1 Drumstk	61	140	13	4	9	2	54.36	75	422	0	0		0.72		
Popcorn, Larger	6 Oz	170	620	30	36	40	10	57.69	73	1046	0	0	20	0.72	0	0
Thigh, Extra Crispy	1 Thigh	118	380	21	14	27	7	63.45	118	625	1	0	20	1.08		
Thigh, Original Recipe	1 Thigh	91	250	16	6	18	4.50	64.80	95	747	1	0	20	0.72		
Whole Wing, Extra Crispy	1 Wing	55	220	10	10	15	4	62.79	55	415	1	0		0.36		
Whole Wing, Original	1 Wing	47	140	9	5	10	2.50	61.64	55	414	0	0		0.36	0	
Crispy Chicken Strips	3 Strips	115	300	26	18	16	4	45	56	1165	1	1		1.08	100	
Pot Pie, Chunky Chicken	13 Oz	368	770	29	69	42	13	49.09	70	2160	5	8	100	1.80	4000	1.20
KFC – Sandwiches																
Chicken, Tender Roast, w/o Sauce	1 Sndwch	177	270	31	26	5	1.50	16.48	65	690	1	1	40	1.80		
Chicken, Triple Crunch w/o Sauce	1 Sndwch	176	390	25	39	15	4.50	34.53	50	650	2	0	40	2.70		

Source: The NutriBase Nutrition Facts Desk Reference. 2nd ed. Avery, a member of Penguin Putnam, Inc. Copyright © 2001 by CyberSoft.

	Serving Size	Gram Weight	Calories (kcals)	Protein (g)	Carbohydrate (g)	Total Fat (g)	Saturated Fat (g)	% kcal from Fat	Cholesterol (mg)	Sodium (mg)	Fiber (g)	Sugars (g)	Calcium (mg)	Iron (mg)	Vitamin A (IU)	Vitamin C (mg)
KFC – Desserts/Snacks																
Cake, Double Choc Chip	1 Serving	76	320	4	41	16	4	44.44	55	230	1	28	40	1.80	0	0
Little Bckt Parfait, Choc Crm	1 Serving	113	290	3	37	15	11	45.76	15	330	2	25	40	1.08		0
Pie, Apple	1 Slice	113	310	2	44	14	3	40.65	0	280	0	23	0	1.08	0	0
Pie, Pecan	1 Slice	113	490	5	66	23	5	42.16	65	510	2	31	20	1.44	200	0
Pie, Strawberry Creme	1 Slice	78	280	4	32	15	8	48.39	15	130	2	22	0	0.72	100	2.40
McDonald's – Breakfast																
Biscuit, Bacon, Egg & Cheese	1 Sndwch	168	540	21	36	34	10	57.30	250	1550	1	4	200	2.70	500	
Biscuit, Sausage w/Egg	1 Sndwch	178	550	18	35	37	10	61.10	245	1160	1	3	100	2.70	300	
Burrito, Breakfast	1 Serving	117	320	13	21	20	7	56.96	195	660	1	2	150	1.80	500	9
Egg McMuffin	1 Sndwch	136	290	17	27	12	4.50	38.03	235	790	1	3	200	2.70	500	1.20
Hash Browns	1 Serving	53	130	1	14	8	1.50	54.55	0	330	1	0		0.36		2.40
Sausage w/Egg McMuffin,	1 Sndwch	162	440	19	27	28	10	57.80	255	890	1	3	250	2.70	500	
Spanish Omelette Bagel	1 Sndwch	258	690	27	59	38	14	49.85	275	1560	10	10	250	4.50	750	15
McDonald's – Chicken																
Chicken McNuggets,	6 Piece	108	290	15	20	17	3.50	52.22	55	540	2	0	20	0.72		
McDonald's – Sandwiches																
Crispy Chicken	1 Sndwch	234	550	23	54	27	4.50	44.10	50	1180	2	7	200	3.60	300	6
Filet-O-Fish	1 Sndwch	156	470	15	45	26	5	49.37	50	890	1	5	200	1.80	200	
McDonald's – Beverages And Shakes																
McFlurry, Oreo,	1 Serving	337	570	15	82	20	12	31.69	70	280	0	69	450	1.08	1250	2.40
Milkshake, Chocolate, Lg.	22 Fl Oz	458	582	15.57	93.89	16.95	10.59	25.64	59.54	444	3.66	81	518	1.42	426	1.83

McDonald's - Burgers

Cheeseburger	1 Burger	121	320	16	35	13	6	36.45	40	830	2	7	250	2.70	300	2.40
Cheeseburger, Qrtr. Pounder	1 Burger	200	530	28	38	30	13	50.56	95	1310	2	9	350	4.50	500	2.40
Hamburger	1 Burger	107	270	13	35	8	3.50	27.27	30	600	2	7	200	2.70	300	2.40
Hamburger, Big Mac	1 Burger	216	570	26	45	32	10	50.35	85	1100	3	8	250	4.50	300	3.60
Hamburger, Qrtr. Pounder	1 Burger	172	430	23	37	21	8	44.06	70	840	2	8	200	4.50	100	2.40
French Fries, Medium	1 Serving	147	450	6	57	22	4	44	0	290	5	0	20	1.08		18

McDonald's - Salads

Chef	1 Salad	206	150	17	5	8	3.50	45	95	740	2	2	150	1.44	1500	15
Garden	1 Salad	149	100	7	4	6	3	55.10	75	120	2	1	150	1.08	1500	15
Grilled Chicken Caesar	1 Salad	163	100	17	3	2.50	1.50	21.95	40	240	2	1	100	1.08	1250	12

McDonald's - Desserts And Snacks

Cookie, Choc. Chip	1 Serving	35	170	2	22	10	6	48.39	20	120	1	13	20	1.08	200	
Ice Cream, Vanilla, Low Fat	1 Serving	90	150	4	23	4.50	3	27.27	20	75	0	17	100	0.36	300	1.20
Pie, Baked Apple	1 Serving	77	260	3	34	13	3.50	44.15	0	200	0	13	20	1.08		24
Sundae, Hot Fudge	1 Serving	179	340	8	52	12	9	31.03	30	170	1	47	250	0.72	500	1.20

Pizza Hut - Pasta

Cavatini Pasta	1 Serving	357	480	21	66	14	6	26.58	8	1170	9	12	150	3.60	1250	
Cavatini Supreme Pasta	1 Serving	396	560	24	73	19	8	30.59	10	1400	10	11	150	4.50	1500	
Spaghetti w/Marinara Sauce	1 Serving	473	490	18	91	6	1	11.02	0	730	8	10	150	3.60	1000	
Spaghetti w/Meat Sauce	1 Serving	467	600	23	98	13	5	19.47	8	910	9	10	100	3.60	1750	

Pizza Hut - Pizza, Medium

Cheese, Hand Tossed	1 Slice	103	309	14	43	9	4.80	26.21	11	848	3.40	8	190	1.26	450	2.40
Cheese, Pan	1 Slice	111	361	13	44	15	5.70	37.19	11	678	3.30	1	200	2.52	500	2.40
Cheese, Thin & Crispy	1 Slice	79	243	11	27	10	4.90	37.19	11	653	2.40	1	190	1.26	450	2.40
Chicken Supreme Pizza, Hand Tossed	1 Slice	116	291	15	44	6	3	18.62	17	841	3.50	9	120	1.26	400	6
Chicken Supreme, Pan	1 Slice	125	343	15	45	12	3.90	31.03	16	671	3.40	2	150	2.70	400	6

Source: The NutriBase Nutrition Facts Desk Reference. 2nd ed. Avery, a member of Penguin Putnam, Inc. Copyright © 2001 by CyberSoft.

Pizza Hut - Pizza, Medium (continued)

	Serving Size	Gram Weight	Calories (kcals)	Protein (g)	Carbohydrate (g)	Total Fat (g)	Saturated Fat (g)	% kcal from Fat	Cholesterol (mg)	Sodium (mg)	Fiber (g)	Sugars (g)	Calcium (mg)	Iron (mg)	Vitamin A (IU)	Vitamin C (mg)
Chicken Supreme Pizza																
Thin & Crispy,	1 Slice	102	232	13	29	7	3.20	27.27	19	681	2.50	2	120	1.44	400	7.20
Meat Lover's Pizza,																
Thin & Crispy	1 Slice	107	339	15	28	19	7.80	49.85	35	970	2.60	1	140	1.80	450	2.40
Meat Lover's, Hand Tossed	1 Slice	121	376	17	44	15	6.40	35.62	30	1077	3.60	8	140	1.62	400	2.40
Meat Lover's, Pan	1 Slice	129	428	16	45	21	7.30	43.65	29	607	3.40	1	140	2.88	450	2.40
Pepperoni, Hand Tossed	1 Slice	100	301	13	43	8	4	24.32	15	867	3.20	8	120	1.26	350	2.40
Pepperoni, Pan	1 Slice	106	353	12	44	14	4.80	36	14	697	3.10	1	130	2.52	350	2.40
Pepperoni, Thin & Crispy	1 Slice	74	235	10	27	10	4.10	37.82	14	672	2.10	1	120	1.26	350	2.40
Supreme, Hand Tossed	1 Slice	123	333	15	44	11	4.90	29.55	18	927	3.70	9	130	1.62	400	6
Supreme, Pan	1 Slice	130	385	14	45	17	5.70	39.33	18	757	3.60	1	140	2.88	400	6
Supreme, Thin & Crispy	1 Slice	110	284	13	29	13	5.50	41.05	20	784	2.80	2	130	1.62	400	16.80
Veggie Lover's, Hand Tossed	1 Slice	120	281	12	45	6	3	19.15	7	771	3.80	9	130	1.44	450	9.60
Veggie Lover's, Pan	1 Slice	125	333	11	46	12	3.90	32.14	7	601	3.60	2	130	2.88	450	9.60
Pizza Hut - Desserts And Snacks																
Apple Dessert Pizza	1 Slice	81	250	3	48	4.50	1	16.56	0	230	2	25		1.08		
Cherry Dessert Pizza	1 Slice	81	250	3	47	4.50	1	16.84	0	220	3	24		1.44	450	
Pizza Hut - Bread																
Bread Stick	1 Serving	38	130	3	20	4	1	28.13	0	170	1	1		1.08		
Bread, Garlic	1 Slice	37	150	3	16	8	1.50	48.65	0	240	1	1	40	1.44	500	

Source: The NutriBase Nutrition Facts Desk Reference. 2nd ed. Avery, a member of Penguin Putnam, Inc. Copyright © 2001 by CyberSoft.

Fitness and Weight Training

In this section of the Behavior Change Log Book you can evaluate your fitness levels, establish fitness goals, and create an overall fitness plan. The following logs will help you track and analyze your cardiorespiratory fitness, weight training, and flexibility programs.

Benefits of Fitness

When evaluating your current fitness levels and prescribing a new exercise regimen, take into account the benefits specific to cardiorespiratory fitness, muscular strength and endurance, and flexibility. Cardiorespiratory fitness decreases the risk of heart disease and diabetes, lowers blood pressure, increases bone density, and contributes to a longer life. Increased muscular strength and endurance lowers the incidence of low back pain, reduces the risk of injuries, reduces the risk of osteoporosis, and improves personal appearance and self-esteem. Improved flexibility results in increased joint mobility, resistance to muscle injury, prevention of low back problems, efficient body movement, and improved posture and personal appearance. By improving all three areas of fitness you will reap the benefits of increased health and wellness, and reduce your risk for many diseases and injuries.

Fitness Goals

Before creating your cardiorespiratory fitness, weight training, and flexibility programs remember that it is important to set goals. Recall from the Changing Behavior section that goals give you something to strive for and serve as motivation for success. Goals should be both specific and realistic. Use the following lines to write down your short-term and long-term goals, target dates for completion, and rewards.

My cardiorespiratory fitness/weight training/flexibility goal is to _____

(long-term goal)

The short-term goals I have established, the deadlines that I have set for them, and the rewards I will receive upon completion are as follows:

_____	_____	_____
(short-term goal 1)	(target date)	(reward)
_____	_____	_____
(short-term goal 2)	(target date)	(reward)
_____	_____	_____
(short-term goal 3)	(target date)	(reward)

My deadline to achieve my long-term goal is _____. The reward I will give

(date)

myself upon realizing my goal is _____

(reward)

Fitness Levels

Determine your current fitness levels using the following tests. You may compare your fitness levels now (preprogram assessment) with your fitness levels after several months of your fitness program (postprogram assessment). For information on performing and evaluating these tests see Chapter 2 of *Total Fitness and Wellness*, Third edition, by Scott K. Powers and Stephen L. Dodd.

Activity	Preprogram Assessment	Postprogram Assessment
Cardiorespiratory Endurance		
1.5-Mile Run Test	_____ time _____ HR	_____ time _____ HR
1-Mile Walk Test	_____ time _____ HR	_____ time _____ HR
Cycle Ergometer Test	_____ time _____ HR	_____ time _____ HR
Step Test	_____ time _____ HR	_____ time _____ HR
Muscular Strength and Endurance		
1 RM (One-Repetition Maximum) Test		
Leg Press	_____ 1 RM (pounds)	_____ 1 RM (pounds)
Bench Press	_____ 1 RM (pounds)	_____ 1 RM (pounds)
Bicep Curl	_____ 1 RM (pounds)	_____ 1 RM (pounds)
Shoulder Press	_____ 1 RM (pounds)	_____ 1 RM (pounds)
Push-up Test	_____ in 60 seconds	_____ in 60 seconds
Sit-up Test	_____ in 60 seconds	_____ in 60 seconds
Curl-up Test	_____ in 75 seconds	_____ in 75 seconds
Flexibility		
Sit and Reach Test	_____ inches	_____ inches
Shoulder Flexibility Test	_____ inches	_____ inches

Exercise Prescriptions

Develop exercise prescriptions for cardiorespiratory fitness, weight training, and flexibility. Build your prescriptions using starter, slow progression, and maintenance phases.

Cardiorespiratory Fitness Prescription

Week No.	Phase	Exercise	Duration (min/day)	Intensity (% of HR_{max})	Frequency (days/wk)	Comments
1						
2						
3						
4						
5						
6						
7						
8						
9						
10						
11						
12						
13						
14						
15						
16						
17						
18						
19						
20						
21						
22						
23						
24						

Weight Training Prescription

Week No.	Phase	Exercise	Weight	Sets/Reps	Frequency (days/wk)	Comments
1						
2						
3						
4						
5						
6						
7						
8						
9						
10						
11						
12						
13						
14						
15						
16						
17						
18						
19						
20						
21						
22						
23						
24						
25						
26						
27						
28						

Flexibility Prescription

Week No.	Exercise	Sets/Hold Time	Frequency (days/wk)	Comments
1				
2				
3				
4				
5				
6				
7				
8				
9				
10				
11				
12				
13				
14				
15				
16				
17				
18				
19				
20				
21				
22				
23				
24				
25				
26				
27				
28				

Exercise Logs

Now, using your exercise prescriptions as guides, log your progress in your new cardiorespiratory, weight training, and flexibility programs.

Cardiorespiratory Fitness Log

DIRECTIONS: In the spaces below keep a record of your cardiorespiratory fitness program. Exercise heart rate can be recorded as the range of heart rates measured at various times during the training session.

Date	Activity	Exercise Duration	Exercise Heart Rate	Comments

Cardiorespiratory Fitness Log

Date	Activity	Exercise Duration	Exercise Heart Rate	Comments

Cardiorespiratory Fitness Log

Date	Activity	Exercise Duration	Exercise Heart Rate	Comments

Cardiorespiratory Fitness Log

Date	Activity	Exercise Duration	Exercise Heart Rate	Comments

Cardiorespiratory Fitness Log

Date	Activity	Exercise Duration	Exercise Heart Rate	Comments

Cardiorespiratory Fitness Log

Date	Activity	Exercise Duration	Exercise Heart Rate	Comments

Weight Training Log

DIRECTIONS: In the spaces below, record the date, number of sets, number of reps, and the weight for each exercise in your weight training program.

Date							
Exercise	St/Rp/Wt	St/Rp/Wt	St/Rp/Wt	St/Rp/Wt	St/Rp/Wt	St/Rp/Wt	St/Rp/Wt

Date							
Exercise	St/Rp/Wt	St/Rp/Wt	St/Rp/Wt	St/Rp/Wt	St/Rp/Wt	St/Rp/Wt	St/Rp/Wt

Weight Training Log

Date							
Exercise	St/Rp/Wt	St/Rp/Wt	St/Rp/Wt	St/Rp/Wt	St/Rp/Wt	St/Rp/Wt	St/Rp/Wt

Date							
Exercise	St/Rp/Wt	St/Rp/Wt	St/Rp/Wt	St/Rp/Wt	St/Rp/Wt	St/Rp/Wt	St/Rp/Wt

Weight Training Log

Date							
Exercise	St/Rp/Wt	St/Rp/Wt	St/Rp/Wt	St/Rp/Wt	St/Rp/Wt	St/Rp/Wt	St/Rp/Wt

Date							
Exercise	St/Rp/Wt	St/Rp/Wt	St/Rp/Wt	St/Rp/Wt	St/Rp/Wt	St/Rp/Wt	St/Rp/Wt

Weight Training Log

Date							
Exercise	St/Rp/Wt	St/Rp/Wt	St/Rp/Wt	St/Rp/Wt	St/Rp/Wt	St/Rp/Wt	St/Rp/Wt

Date							
Exercise	St/Rp/Wt	St/Rp/Wt	St/Rp/Wt	St/Rp/Wt	St/Rp/Wt	St/Rp/Wt	St/Rp/Wt

Weight Training Log

Date							
Exercise	St/Rp/Wt	St/Rp/Wt	St/Rp/Wt	St/Rp/Wt	St/Rp/Wt	St/Rp/Wt	St/Rp/Wt

Date							
Exercise	St/Rp/Wt	St/Rp/Wt	St/Rp/Wt	St/Rp/Wt	St/Rp/Wt	St/Rp/Wt	St/Rp/Wt

Weight Training Log

Date							
Exercise	St/Rp/Wt	St/Rp/Wt	St/Rp/Wt	St/Rp/Wt	St/Rp/Wt	St/Rp/Wt	St/Rp/Wt

Date							
Exercise	St/Rp/Wt	St/Rp/Wt	St/Rp/Wt	St/Rp/Wt	St/Rp/Wt	St/Rp/Wt	St/Rp/Wt

Weight Training Log

Date							
Exercise	St/Rp/Wt	St/Rp/Wt	St/Rp/Wt	St/Rp/Wt	St/Rp/Wt	St/Rp/Wt	St/Rp/Wt

Date							
Exercise	St/Rp/Wt	St/Rp/Wt	St/Rp/Wt	St/Rp/Wt	St/Rp/Wt	St/Rp/Wt	St/Rp/Wt

Weight Training Log

Date							
Exercise	St/Rp/Wt	St/Rp/Wt	St/Rp/Wt	St/Rp/Wt	St/Rp/Wt	St/Rp/Wt	St/Rp/Wt

Date							
Exercise	St/Rp/Wt	St/Rp/Wt	St/Rp/Wt	St/Rp/Wt	St/Rp/Wt	St/Rp/Wt	St/Rp/Wt

Weight Training Log

Date							
Exercise	St/Rp/Wt	St/Rp/Wt	St/Rp/Wt	St/Rp/Wt	St/Rp/Wt	St/Rp/Wt	St/Rp/Wt

Date							
Exercise	St/Rp/Wt	St/Rp/Wt	St/Rp/Wt	St/Rp/Wt	St/Rp/Wt	St/Rp/Wt	St/Rp/Wt

Weight Training Log

Date							
Exercise	St/Rp/Wt	St/Rp/Wt	St/Rp/Wt	St/Rp/Wt	St/Rp/Wt	St/Rp/Wt	St/Rp/Wt

Date							
Exercise	St/Rp/Wt	St/Rp/Wt	St/Rp/Wt	St/Rp/Wt	St/Rp/Wt	St/Rp/Wt	St/Rp/Wt

Flexibility Log

DIRECTIONS: In the spaces below, record the date, sets, and hold time for each exercise in your flexibility program.

Date							
Exercise	St/Hold	St/Hold	St/Hold	St/Hold	St/Hold	St/Hold	St/Hold

Date							
Exercise	St/Hold	St/Hold	St/Hold	St/Hold	St/Hold	St/Hold	St/Hold

Flexibility Log

Date							
Exercise	St/Hold	St/Hold	St/Hold	St/Hold	St/Hold	St/Hold	St/Hold

Date							
Exercise	St/Hold	St/Hold	St/Hold	St/Hold	St/Hold	St/Hold	St/Hold

Flexibility Log

Date							
Exercise	St/Hold	St/Hold	St/Hold	St/Hold	St/Hold	St/Hold	St/Hold

Date							
Exercise	St/Hold	St/Hold	St/Hold	St/Hold	St/Hold	St/Hold	St/Hold

Flexibility Log

Date							
Exercise	St/Hold	St/Hold	St/Hold	St/Hold	St/Hold	St/Hold	St/Hold

Date							
Exercise	St/Hold	St/Hold	St/Hold	St/Hold	St/Hold	St/Hold	St/Hold

Flexibility Log

Date							
Exercise	St/Hold	St/Hold	St/Hold	St/Hold	St/Hold	St/Hold	St/Hold

Date							
Exercise	St/Hold	St/Hold	St/Hold	St/Hold	St/Hold	St/Hold	St/Hold

Flexibility Log

Date							
Exercise	St/Hold	St/Hold	St/Hold	St/Hold	St/Hold	St/Hold	St/Hold

Date							
Exercise	St/Hold	St/Hold	St/Hold	St/Hold	St/Hold	St/Hold	St/Hold

Wellness Journal Topics

As you study health and wellness issues in your class, you may find that you wish to explore your ideas and feelings on the topics further. Use the suggested journal topics in this section as a starting point for investigation into your health and healthy behavior.

1 Taking Responsibility for Healthy Behavior Change

Are you as healthy as you would like to be? What are some obstacles that may be keeping you from attaining optimal health? What are you hoping to learn in this class that will change your health behavior in the future?

2 Psychosocial Health: Mental, Emotional, Social, and Spiritual Wellness

Ways to enhance psychosocial health include getting enough sleep, developing self-esteem, and having a spiritual connection with the world. Do you feel especially strong or weak in any of these areas? What steps can you take to improve your psychosocial health?

3 Managing Stress

Think about the major stressors in your life: classes, work, relationships, and so on. What is a concrete step you can take now to cope with one aspect of the most significant stressor? For example, you might need to improve your time management skills or practice more assertive communication. Follow the strategy for a week, then evaluate your stress level again.

4 Coping with Violence and Unintentional Injuries

Consider the effects that violence has had on your life, either as a direct victim or witness of it, or indirectly through depictions of violence in the media and elsewhere. How did you cope with a particular event? How would you advise others to respond?

5 Healthy Relationships

Think about healthy and unhealthy relationships in your life. Identify some of the differences between the two types. Are your communication patterns the same in both relationships? What is the role of factors such as age, gender, and culture on the success or failure of these relationships?

6 Sexuality: Making Healthy Choices

How did you learn about sexual behavior and sexual orientation? Parents? Friends? School? Were your questions answered? Was the information accurate? Do you think these learning experiences affected your feelings about sexuality positively or negatively?

7 Reproductive Choices: Contraception and Planning a Family

If you chose to be sexually active, what steps would you take to obtain and use contraception? Make a list of the methods you would consider and list the pros and cons of each method.

8 Nutrition: Eating Smart

Keep track of everything that you eat and drink for one week, then compare it to the Food Guide Pyramid. Which groups are you most likely to eat more of than the recommended servings? Which groups do you eat less of than recommended? What is the impact of these patterns on your health?

9 Managing Your Weight

Do you eat because it's time to eat, or because you are really hungry? Record your eating behaviors for three days. Each time you find yourself eating or drinking, ask yourself whether you are really hungry and what triggered you to eat.

10 Getting and Staying Fit

How do you define physical fitness? Does it include appearance, endurance, heart rate, or other factors? How does this compare to the definition presented in your health class? Which components are the most motivating to you to start or continue a fitness program?

11 Addictions and Addictive Behavior

Have you ever had a habit that you tried and failed to break? Would you consider it an addiction? What do you think the difference is between a habit and an addiction?

12 Using Alcohol Responsibly

Keep a record of your alcohol use over the next two weeks. Were there any times when you drank when you hadn't planned to or drank more than you meant to? What led to these situations? What are some strategies that can help you manage your drinking responsibly in the future?

13 Tobacco

Think about the people you know who are tobacco users (and yourself if you use tobacco). Why do you think they started? What are the biggest obstacles facing them when they try to quit?

14 Illicit Drugs

Consider the drug education programs that you were exposed to in elementary, junior high, and high school. Were any of them effective? If so, why? If not, how would you design a more effective program?

15 Cardiovascular Disease: Risk Reduction

Think about the strategies you have learned for preventing cardiovascular disease. Which are you most likely to put into practice? If you implement a strategy such as weight management or stopping smoking, do you think the short-term or long-term benefits will be more motivating for you?

16 Cancer: Understanding Your Risks

What types of cancers do you think you and your friends are at greatest risk for right now? Are you doing anything to reduce your risk? If so, what? If not, why not?

17 Sexually Transmitted Infections and Other Infectious Diseases

List the ways in which you have protected yourself from catching an STI or other infectious disease. Which were easy to do and which were more difficult? Are you likely to continue the same behaviors in the future?

18 Noninfectious Diseases

How much individual responsibility should we each accept for chronic diseases we could have prevented? Do you have any lifestyle or personal health habits such as smoking or being overweight that could contribute to a chronic disease? Have you tried to change any of these habits?

19 Healthy Aging

Picture yourself reaching retirement age. What are you doing now to ensure that you are as healthy and secure as you picture yourself being?

20 Dying and Death

Describe how you would like your funeral or memorial service to be. Who would speak at it? What do you hope people would say about you?

21 Living in a Healthy Environment

Of the many ways that you can contribute to a healthier environment (recycling, picking up litter, writing legislators), which are you the most likely to do consistently? Do you think it is more important that your actions have an immediate or long-term impact?

22 Being a Smart Healthcare Consumer

Learn about your own insurance protection. What coverage do you currently have? If you don't have coverage, how would you pay for a medical emergency? What coverage is available to you as a student? What is covered and not covered by your insurance plan?

23 Complementary and Alternative Medicine (CAM)

Among the most common CAM practices are chiropractic treatments, acupuncture, and herbal remedies. If a friend used one of these treatments instead of a traditional medical treatment for a condition, would your response be positive, negative, or neutral? Would you advise your friend to ask more or different questions of the practitioners? Would your expectations for the outcome be the same?

Behavior Change Contract

DIRECTIONS: Choose a health behavior that you would like to change, starting this quarter or semester (see page 125 for a sample filled-in contract). Sign the contract at the bottom to affirm your commitment to making a healthy change and ask a friend to witness it.

My behavior change will be:

_____

My long-term goal for this behavior change is:

_____

These are three obstacles to change (things that I am currently doing or situations that contribute to this behavior or make it harder to change):

1. _____

2. _____

3. _____

The strategies I will use to overcome these obstacles are:

1. _____

2. _____

3. _____

Resources I will use to help me change this behavior include:

a friend/partner/relative: _____

_____

a school-based resource: _____

_____

a community-based resource: _____

_____

a book or reputable website: _____

_____

In order to make my goal more attainable, I have devised these short-term goals.

short-term goal	target date	reward

short-term goal	target date	reward

short-term goal	target date	reward

When I make the long-term behavior change described above, my reward will be:

_____   Target date: _____

I intend to make the behavior change described above. I will use the strategies and rewards to achieve the goals that will contribute to a healthy behavior change.

Signed: _____   Witness: _____

Sample Behavior Change Contract

DIRECTIONS: Choose a health behavior that you would like to change, starting this quarter or semester. Sign the contract at the bottom to affirm your commitment to making a healthy change and ask a friend to witness it.

My behavior change will be:

To snack less on junk food and more on healthy foods

My long-term goal for this behavior change is:

Eat junk food snacks no more than once a week

These are three obstacles to change (things that I am currently doing or situations that contribute to this behavior or make it harder to change):

1. *The grocery store is closed by the time I come home from school*

2. *I get hungry between classes and the vending machines only carry candy bars*

3. *It's easier to order pizza or other snacks than to make a snack at home*

The strategies I will use to overcome these obstacles are:

1. *I'll leave early for school once a week so I can stock up on healthy snacks in the morning*

2. *I'll bring a piece of fruit or other healthy snack to eat between classes*

3. *I'll learn some easy recipes for snacks to make at home*

Resources I will use to help me change this behavior include:

a friend/partner/relative: *My roommates: I'll ask them to buy healthier snacks instead of chips when they do the shopping*

a school-based resource: *The dining hall: I'll ask the manager to provide healthy foods we can take to eat between classes*

a community-based resource: *The library: I'll check out some cookbooks to find easy snack ideas*

a book or reputable website: *The USDA nutrient database at www.nal.usda.gov/fnic: I'll use this site to make sure the foods I select are healthy choices*

In order to make my goal more attainable, I have devised these short-term goals.

Eat a healthy snack 3 times per week	*September 15*	*New CD*
short-term goal	target date	reward
Learn to make a healthy snack	*October 15*	*Concert ticket*
short-term goal	target date	reward
Eat a healthy snack 5 times per week	*November 15*	*New shoes*
short-term goal	target date	reward

When I make the long-term behavior change described above, my reward will be:

Ski lift tickets for winter break   Target date: *December 15*

I intend to make the behavior change described above. I will use the strategies and rewards to achieve the goals that will contribute to a healthy behavior change.

Signed: *Elizabeth King*   Witness: *Susan Bauer*

Lifelong Behavior Change Contract

DIRECTIONS: Behavior change is a process that continues for a lifetime. The strategies that you begin to follow now can contribute to healthy benefits far into the future. Choose a change that will have long-term positive effects, then complete the contract and put your intentions into action (see page 129 for a sample filled-in contract). Sign the contract at the bottom to affirm your commitment to making a healthy change and ask a friend to witness it.

My behavior change will be:

_____

My long-term goal for this behavior change is:

_____

These are three obstacles to change (things that I am currently doing or situations that contribute to this behavior or make it harder to change):

1. _____

2. _____

3. _____

The strategies I will use to overcome these obstacles are:

1. _____

2. _____

3. _____

Resources I will use to help me change this behavior include:

a friend/partner/relative: _____

a school-based resource: _____

a community-based resource: _____

a book or reputable website: _____

In order to make my goal more attainable, I have devised these short-term goals.

_____   _____   _____
short-term goal   target date   reward

_____   _____   _____
short-term goal   target date   reward

_____   _____   _____
short-term goal   target date   reward

When I make the long-term behavior change described above, my reward will be:

_____   Target date: _____

I intend to make the behavior change described above. I will use the strategies and rewards to achieve the goals that will contribute to a healthy behavior change.

Signed: _____ Witness: _____

Sample Lifelong Behavior Change Contract

DIRECTIONS: Behavior change is a process that continues for a lifetime. The strategies that you begin to follow now can contribute to healthy benefits far into the future. Choose a change that will have long-term positive effects, then complete the contract and put your intentions into action. Sign the contract at the bottom to affirm your commitment to making a healthy change and ask a friend to witness it.

My behavior change will be:

To incorporate exercise into my daily life

My long-term goal for this behavior change is:

To maintain a healthy weight and feel fit

These are three obstacles to change (things that I am currently doing or situations that contribute to this behavior or make it harder to change):

1. *I get bored doing the same exercise all of the time*

2. *I find myself watching TV I don't even enjoy and then not having time to exercise*

3. *I'm afraid I'll injure myself doing new activities*

The strategies I will use to overcome these obstacles are:

1. *I'll learn several activities so that I have variety in my exercise program*

2. *I'll give myself a set number of "TV hours" and use the extra time for exercise*

3. *I'll get a complete check-up with my physician before I start a new exercise program*

Resources I will use to help me change this behavior include:

a friend/partner/relative: *I'll ask friends to exercise with me so I stay motivated and don't get bored*

a school-based resource: *I'll find out what types of activities are offered by the PE department*

a community-based resource: *I'll join a local club that does the activity I enjoy most*

a book or reputable website: *I'll track my progress in the Fitness section of my Log Book and Wellness Journal*

In order to make my goal more attainable, I have devised these short-term goals.

Walk to school three times a week	_3 months from today_	_dinner out at my favorite restaurant_
short-term goal	target date	reward
Learn a new activity to add to my exercise program	_6 months from today_	_new outfit_
short-term goal	target date	reward
Participate in the local 10k walk/run	_1 year from today_	_weekend vacation_
short-term goal	target date	reward

When I make the long-term behavior change described above, my reward will be:

vacation trip   Target date: _2 years from now_

I intend to make the behavior change described above. I will use the strategies and rewards to achieve the goals that will contribute to a healthy behavior change.

Signed: _Barry Snow_   Witness: _Rob Santiago_

References

Access to Health
Eighth Edition
By Rebecca J. Donatelle
ISBN 0-8053-5564-2

Decisions for Healthy Living
By B.E. Pruitt and Jane J. Stein
ISBN 0-321-10671-7

DINE Systems, Inc.
586 N. French Road
Amherst, NY 14228
716-688-2492
FAX 716-688-2505

Health The Basics
Fifth Edition
By Rebecca J. Donatelle
ISBN 0-8053-5326-7

NutriFit CD-ROM
Developed by NutriBase.com
in partnership with Benjamin Cummings Publishing
ISBN 0-321-11218-0
To order call 1-800-282-0693
or e-mail PearsonEd@eds.com

Total Fitness and Wellness
Third Edition
By Scott K. Powers and Stephen L. Dodd
ISBN 0-205-34095-4
To order call 1-800-282-0693
or e-mail PearsonEd@eds.com